ADAPTED PHYSICAL EDUCATION
FOR
STUDENTS WITH AUTISM

ADAPTED PHYSICAL EDUCATION
FOR
STUDENTS WITH AUTISM

By

KIMBERLY DAVIS, M.S. (Physical Education)

Specialization in Adapted Physical Education
Indiana University
Institute for the Study of Developmental Disabilities
Adapted Physical Education Specialist Consultant

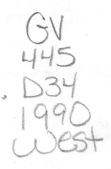

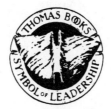

CHARLES C THOMAS • PUBLISHER
Springfield • Illinois • U.S.A.

Published and Distributed Throughout the World by

CHARLES C THOMAS • PUBLISHER
2600 South First Street
Springfield, Illinois 62794-9265

© *1990 by* CHARLES C THOMAS • PUBLISHER

ISBN 0-398-05688-9

Library of Congress Catalog Card Number: 90-33488

With THOMAS BOOKS *careful attention is given to all details of manufacturing
and design. It is the Publisher's desire to present books that are satisfactory as to their
physical qualities and artistic possibilities and appropriate for their particular use.*
THOMAS BOOKS *will be true to those laws of quality that assure a good name
and good will.*

Printed in the United States of America
SC-R-3

Library of Congress Cataloging-in-Publication Data

Davis, Kimberly
   Adapted physical education for students with autism / by Kimberly
Davis.
      p. cm.
   Includes bibliographical references.
   ISBN 0-398-05688-9
   1. Physical education for handicapped children.   2. Autistic
children.   I. Title.
GV445.D34   1990
613.7'042—dc20

90-33488
CIP

This book is dedicated to
Heather
for helping me form my views of seeing
abilities rather than disabilities,
possibilities rather than impossibilities,
and
love rather than indifference.

PREFACE

This volume is the culmination of eight years of work in a research and development center for children and youth with autism at Indiana University. The program which provided the basis for this manuscript was established to help students begin to learn basic gross motor skills which could then be carried over to play/leisure time activities. Communication, integration, and independence of movement were all stressed as major goals of the program. The suggestions herein are the author's attempt to assist her colleagues in the field who may encounter students with autism or similar problems with communication and social interaction.

ACKNOWLEDGMENTS

I wish to extend my appreciation to Dr. Susan K. Shuster and Georgia Sheriff for their enthusiasm and encouragement, and time to complete this text while on the job. Thanks to Nancy Dalrymple for her expertise in autism and her comments regarding the text.

Special thanks to Stine Levy, Annamaria Mecca, and Barbara Porco, my colleagues on the Autism/Assessment Training Team at the Institute, for their written and spoken comments, critical reading, encouragement, and the expert knowledge they shared with me over the years.

INTRODUCTION

This book has been written for physical educators and adapted physical educators who may encounter children or young adults with autism. Autism is a severe communication disorder which is life long. People with autism also have great difficulties in daily social interaction. Most people with autism are also retarded to some degree, yet some may have normal or above normal intelligence. The diversity of characteristics of autism creates a unique challenge to educators.

Autism is a very puzzling disorder, which to date has not been discussed in great detail in most adapted physical education texts. In the texts which were reviewed, autism was hidden within the discussion of emotional disturbance. Most frequently the description was a series of paragraphs with very sketchy information or, worse, misinformation about autism. This limited and misleading description of autism is often the only reference undergraduate students receive in their course of study. It is not the author's intent to taint the value of these texts, but to illustrate the need for additional information. This book will describe autism and offer suggestions regarding the assessment and programming for students with autism in adapted physical education/regular physical education classes.

Since physical education is written into P.L. 94-142 as part of the required education of special students, every effort should be made to provide them with a quality education. Proper adapted physical education can often be overlooked as a necessary part of the school day. It is important to keep in mind that physical educators and other teachers working with students with autism must all work together to provide the student with the best possible program. Physical education for special students is often part of a team or interdisciplinary approach. No one discipline can program in isolation. Interdisciplinary approaches increase the flow of ideas and keep morale up, while maximizing the students' level of learning.

CONTENTS

ADAPTED PHYSICAL EDUCATION
FOR
STUDENTS WITH AUTISM

Chapter One

GENERAL OVERVIEW OF AUTISM

Autism is puzzling. The disorder is so puzzling that textbook authors may differ substantially in their descriptions of the disorder. This can lead to confusion among the professionals who encounter and teach students with autism. An understanding of autism, or any other disorder, is needed in order to facilitate proper programs for these students. The following overview is an attempt to unify all of the current information and make it applicable to the physical education teacher.

DEFINITION

Autism, by federal definition, is a developmental disability. This definition emphasizes what a person can or cannot do rather than labeling the disability. The general characteristics of autism which fit the federal definition are one: early onset. With autism this onset is evident in infancy or in childhood (DSM III–R). Secondly, the disability persists throughout the individual's life; it does not go away, nor does the child "outgrow" the autism. It is lifelong. Lastly, the individual's ability to cope with life is greatly affected. More specific to autism is the fact that language development and social development are significantly delayed. The central nervous system of people with autism cannot process all of the sensory stimulation and input that it receives; thus, coping with everyday situations becomes very difficult or impossible without some guidance and teaching.

CAUSES

There are many theories surrounding the causes of autism. Particularly damaging is the theory stating that parents cause their child to become autistic. This is not true. Autism is an organic disorder which affects the central nervous system and interferes with normal development. It manifests itself in a wide range of behavioral symptoms (Coleman and

Gillberg, 1985). Professionals are not able to explain autism with one single cause or set of causes. There are many possible theories which link autism with environmental factors. Exposure of the parents to occupational chemicals such as paint, farm chemicals, or water-treatment chemicals for a prolonged period of time has been noticed in some cases (Coleman and Gillberg, 1985; Felicetti, 1981). Damage to the fetus during pregnancy or bleeding in the middle trimester of pregnancy have also been documented. Genetic factors such as a family history of speech delay, learning disability or other developmental disorders, plus other genetic links to Fragile X syndrome or PKU, have come to the forefront as possible correlates to autism (Coleman and Gillberg, 1985). All of these theories suggest that there is something which affects the child's central nervous system enough to interfere with normal development and cause the child to become very different from other children. No one theory can explain everything about autism. At best they can offer ideas or clues as to what has been damaged and why, but not how to cure it. However, the current researchers are leaning towards a combination of genetic and biological factors.

PREVALENCE

Within the total population autism is relatively rare, affecting 5 to 20 of 10,000 births (Wing and Gould, 1979; Gillberg, 1984). This number is similar to the numbers of children born who are congenitally blind or deaf. Most people are not likely to encounter people with autism in their everyday lives since the numbers are so rare within the total population. Many families with children who have autism note that the general public does not understand or recognize autism. Some families have reported that the police have been called when someone mistakes a tantrum as a response to child abuse. Misinformation or insufficient information can add to this problem. The disability itself is usually not physically visible; thus, uninformed people have no outward clues to help explain the unusual behaviors they may see.

However, within the population of developmentally disabled students the number with autism dramatically increases. Rather than 5–20 in 10,000, the numbers become 1–5 in 20 with autism (Levy, personal communication, 1986). This means that it is very likely that those teachers who work with developmentally disabled students will encounter students with autism in their classes.

MENTAL ABILITIES

The range of intelligence in people with autism contributes to the confusion for professionals. Individuals with autism have IQ scores which range from severely retarded to average or above average. Most do have some degree of retardation. Testing has shown that 60 percent have an IQ below 50, 20 percent between 50–70, and only 20 percent above 70 (Rutter, 1983). That means 80 percent of people with autism also have mental retardation. What adds even more to the puzzle is the fact that some people with autism may show some amazing splinter skills such as recall of complete movie scene dialogues, mathematical abilities such as adding or multiplying large numbers instantaneously, word recall/recognition of new, unrelated words, or extraordinary artistic abilities. These splinter skills can often cause confusion regarding the individual's true mental abilities. Educators, health care providers and others may key into the person's splinter skill and use that one skill as the basis for how much that person knows as a whole. Much of this splinter skill knowledge is fun for the individual but is not functional or useful in everyday living.

Chapter Two

CHARACTERISTICS OF AUTISM

Autism is a difficult disorder to differentiate. Persons with autism are often mistakenly thought to be deaf, severely emotionally disturbed, socially immature, mentally retarded, aphasic, or communication impaired. Autism is often accompanied by many of the characteristics that appear in each of the above-mentioned disorders, but it is the combination and persistence of characteristics which define the autistic syndrome.

What are the characteristics which distinguish autism from other developmental disorders? The following characteristics are listed in the DSM III–R definition of autism:

Onset during infancy or childhood
Qualitative impairment in verbal and nonverbal communication, and in imaginative activity
Qualitative impairment in reciprocal social interaction

To this list I would add the following:

Predictability
Uneven rate of development
Disturbance of sensory system
Variability

These characteristics are important to document when doing an assessment. Each characteristic has important points which must be understood to grasp the total scope of the autistic syndrome.

VARIABILITY

This characteristic will be discussed first because it may be the most important to help understand autism and how its effects are observed in each individual.

When babies are born all begin to react to the world around them in similar ways, i.e., cooing, babbling, moving, looking around, smiling, etc. As they grow and mature, their experiences differ and they become more unique and varied. This is also true of children with autism. The younger they are, the more alike they all appear; as they age, differences become more noticeable.

People who are more severely retarded appear to be more alike than people with higher intelligence in terms of communication skills, social skills, movement, etc. The intelligence of a person greatly affects that person's ability to interact with the environment. Persons with autism who are not also retarded will exhibit more diversity than will those who are retarded. When thinking of people with autism, these two factors, age and IQ, must be considered. The following diagram symbolizes the concept of variability among people with autism.

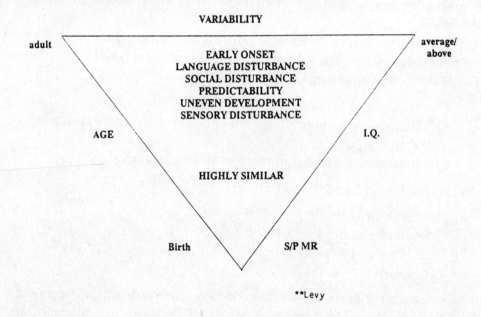

This triangle represents people with autism and lists the characteristics of autism. The top of the triangle indicates the wide degree of variability possible among people with autism and the bottom represents the highly similar aspects. The variability then is affected by age and IQ. The more intelligent and older the person with autism, the more varied he may seem from the person with autism who is not as intelligent. All people with autism should not be lumped together in a "see one, seen them all" box. Just as other people vary and change with age and intelligence, so do people with autism. All individuals with autism share some common characteristics. For all of their lives, young or old, retarded or not, they are always present in varying degrees. Thus each individual is unique, yet they have characteristics in common.

AGE OF ONSET

This is an important characteristic to document in order to distinguish autism from the other disabilities. In order to do this, a developmental history from the child's parents or guardians must be obtained. This focuses on the first 30–36 months of the child's life; not so much on the physical milestones as on the early memories of how the child responded to affection, made needs known, played or interacted with parents, toys, and surroundings. Also, information on how the child reacted to changes and on sensory development are important. Children with autism have some differences from normally developing children which can be picked up during this parent interview (Levy, 1985).

In her study of autism, DeMyer (1979) noted three different times in the child's life when some differences were noticed about the child. The first point of awareness is noticed immediately; the child is different from birth. This can be noticed in one of two ways: the child can be a baby that is "too good to be true" and never a problem. The baby doesn't cry or fuss and can be taken anywhere. This can be overlooked as a problem since the baby does not interfere with daily activities. On the other hand, the baby may be one who cannot be pacified at all. This baby may cry continually without being quieted by food, touch, or movement.

The second point of awareness comes at approximately 18 months of age. The child appears to be developing normally when things suddenly stop, decrease, or drastically change in some way. This is especially noted in the language and social interaction areas. Quite often these changes are tied to an event that the parents remember happening at around the same time. These events are usually something disturbing such as a fight, a death in the family, the birth of another child, or a move to a new location. Parents feel that the child somehow picked up on the change and became so upset that language stopped or the child did not want to interact any more. This is their attempt to understand the reason for the radical change in behavior and to help alleviate any guilt they may feel.

The third point of awareness is gradual and subtle. The child appears to be progressing appropriately with no problems, until suddenly, when other children of the same age are around, differences become quite apparent. The language is not the same, skills may be absent, the play patterns and interactions of the child are not like that of the other children. When compared to the other children in preschool or to a younger sibling, the child with autism stands out. Progress has been very slow or different.

With each of these stages of awareness, the autism has usually been present from birth, but parents notice the differences in their child at various stages of development. Perception of the problem varies with each child and family.

Recent research has indicated that some young children may become autistic after having an illness such as encephalitis or after having a stroke (Gillberg, 1986). Prior to the malady they may have been developing normally, yet the central nervous system insult caused the child to have an arrest in development and develop autism.

QUALITATIVE IMPAIRMENT OF COMMUNICATION

Language and communication skills of people with autism are greatly affected by the disorder. Fifty percent of the people with autism do not learn how to talk; generally, this group of people are moderately to severely retarded as well as autistic. (This group will be referred to as "low functioning" individuals with autism.) Gestures which are used by the general population such as a shoulder shrug to mean "I don't know" are not understood readily by these people. They do not know how to use gestures, such as pointing, to get a desired object or response; often they will take a person to the object instead of simply pointing to that object. There is also little understanding of facial expressions depicting emotions or social cues.

Communication skills can vary from a student with no verbal communication to one who is highly verbal. This can cause confusion for educators and difficulty in programming for these students. Often, the expressive language is echolalic, repeating back what is heard. This echoing may be immediate or may be delayed. This means that the student is not using original language but is repeating something that s/he heard at one time and enjoyed. The language may be an attempt by that student to communicate to the adult in the only way s/he knows how or it may be a form of self-stimulation. Songs or TV commercials are favorites for repeating, as well as greetings which are rehearsed continually in an attempt to communicate.

Receptive language is also difficult for a person with autism. Standard assessments have shown that in many of the people with autism, the level of expressive language is similar to the level of his/her receptive language skills. This may vary if the assessment includes functional understanding and use of language. Also, the intervention, particularly with an augmentative system, would affect this "rule of thumb." These individuals do not necessarily hear all of what is said to them or may take a longer time than usual to process any information said to them. Many times this inability to understand directions or conversations is mistaken for willful disobedience when, in fact, the student simply did not understand what was said. For this reason many of these students are said to be severe behavior problems. This may be true, but the behavior problems are a result of their inability to understand the rules and requirements of their environment. For this reason it is important that the primary focus of treatment/therapy/intervention be communication and that the behavior be a secondary consideration.

Often, the person with autism seems to understand a great deal more than s/he truly does. Teachers, and sometimes parents, believe that the student is being purposefully disobedient rather than not understanding what is being said or what is happening. What might explain the sense that "I know he understands what I want him to do, he just doesn't want to do this"? Prizant and Schuler (1987) offer the following explanations as to what a person with autism may be responding to when he appears to understand spoken language. The student might be responding to (1) a familiar routine, (2) environmental cues such as going to the table when the refrigerator door is opened, (3) high probability events or doing what is usually done such as brushing teeth when given a toothbrush, (4) parts of an utterance, especially the last word or words, and (5) intonation. All too often it can be taken for granted that the student knows exactly what is requested and it is expected that the request will be carried out. When it is not, the student is at fault for not listening or being "bad."

QUALITATIVE IMPAIRMENT IN INTERACTION

People with autism do not relate to people or objects in the way others normally do. Objects or toys can become very special to a person with autism, so much so that the toys can interfere with progress in the child's school program or work in the workshop. Some people can become very attached to strings, stuffed animals, balls or special toys. At times these people can be most reluctant to release these items or their favorite toy even for a second. They do not play with toys in the normally intended manner. Cars may be turned over in order to spin the wheels, blocks may be lined up in a very ritualistic fashion, tricycles tipped over to spin the wheel, or balls tossed only to watch them roll across the floor. Individual play of children with autism is also different. Some children may choose to sit in a rocker with a headband covering their eyes, earphones on and listening to music; another may sit on a mini-trampoline and chew on a teething ring; still another might stand in the corner and feel the wall. Children with autism do not know how to play with toys or how to appropriately entertain themselves.

One of the many myths surrounding autism is that people with autism are not cuddly or are withdrawn when it comes to any interpersonal interactions. Many times these people can become cuddly to a fault and approach adults with no hesitation. Rules or social cues that others learn regarding who can be touched and when it is all right to do so are not integrated by those with autism. Because of this willingness to approach adults, some people choose to believe these individuals do not have autism. People with autism seem to form a simple hierarchy of interaction. Generally, they are most likely to interact with adults, then their siblings, and finally their peers (Levy, 1985). The reason for this hierarchy may be in part due to the need for sameness which people with autism possess. This sameness is evident in adults. Adults are usually consistent and predictable in dealing with others and especially with children. Reactions to situations are generally the same in all adults, whether feeling happy, sad, or angry. Each adult is similar in the reactions evoked and displayed. Brothers and sisters, next on the hierarchy, grow up with this child who is different. They learn the needs of the child with autism and how to respond to them in a fairly consistent manner. They may not always react in the "right" way, but are more consistent than the child's peers. Especially at a young age, children are very unpredictable from moment to moment. They might scream, push, take toys, touch, get too close, or just be "normally" childlike. The "normal" childlike behavior can be too confusing and frightening to a child with autism. There is little predictability with children and their play habits. People with autism crave sameness and strive for it in their day-to-day routines.

These people with autism want to control their environment as much as possible. Changes and unexpected events, such as an unexpected touch or hug, even from an adult, are not always pleasant for a child with autism. Yet, when they choose to hug or touch, it can be fine. Oftentimes, the individual will initiate an "okay" touch or hug. Care must be taken to respect this need and not expect them to react to touch normally, since they are not typical.

PREDICTABILITY

As indicated previously, people with autism are resistant to change. Change is frightening to them. They do not innately understand changes in their daily routine. If they miss breakfast, go a different way to school, or brush their teeth before rather than after breakfast, there may be problems. Many unexpected or unexplained changes can cause behavior problems. Understanding their communication and processing difficulties is important when discussing the need for sameness. Most adults and children can cope fairly well with changes in their day. Getting up late, missing morning coffee, or fire drills can be dealt with in most cases. They can talk about the change with someone or rationalize it themselves. People with autism do not always have the abilities to understand that changes are only temporary and that life will go on as usual. Not knowing what is happening and being pushed and prodded to do a task a different way or to do a new task can be traumatic for some children with autism. For teachers and parents of children with autism the task is to help them understand their daily routine.

This need for sameness will always be present to some degree. It is a mistake to think that as the student becomes familiar with people and surroundings that the need for sameness will disappear. It may decrease somewhat, but it does not go away. They will need a consistent, structured routine to follow throughout their lives in order to function in a semi-independent, acceptable manner. This will be true at home, school, and, finally, work.

It is also important for home, school, and work to keep an open and active line of communication going at all times. Since students with autism do not generalize skills well, all areas need to know what is going on in other environments. Information shared might include expectations per discipline/area, behavior plans being followed, or new skills acquired. Consistency cannot be stressed enough so that the student can learn and many unnecessary behavior problems can be avoided.

UNEVEN RATE OF DEVELOPMENT

All people with autism develop in an uneven manner. When looking at a developmental profile of a person with autism which includes the areas of mental abilities, academics, language skills, motor skills, self-help skills and social and play skills, it becomes obvious that the development is in an uneven pattern.

The following profile is an example of one child's developmental levels.

5 1/2 YR OLD BOY: AUTISM

Note that the score for mental abilities is listed as a nonverbal test. This nonverbal test utilizes visual and fine motor skills as the measure of intelligence. The child's task is to match a character or symbol pattern presented to him/her on blocks. The designs become more intricate and difficult as the test progresses. There is very little talking necessary when administering this test. This is important to realize due to the fact that most tests of mental abilities are verbal tests. Since children with autism have a great difficulty with language, a test which is verbally based would not be testing mental abilities but rather language skills.

The two areas in which all people with autism have the most deficits are in the language area and social/play skills. Generally, the scores for these two areas fall below the scores for mental abilities even if the child is higher functioning. The higher functioning student with autism, those who range from mildly retarded to average or above average intelligence, usually develop some coping mechanisms which help him/her survive in the world. The scores will be uneven. This pattern of low scores in language and social/play skills is typical of people with autism. There are differences when comparing the profile of a student with autism to that of a learning disabled student or a child who is mentally retarded. Figures 3 and 4 illustrate the differences which can be seen in the pattern of scores.

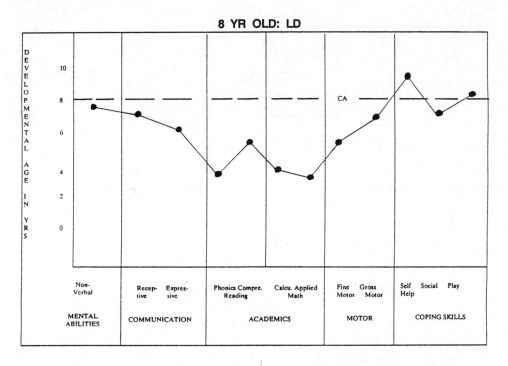

The scores of the student with learning disabilities show problems in academics but not the severe difficulties in language or social and play categories noted in the profile of the student with autism.

The scores of the mentally retarded child are more evenly distributed in all areas. There is not such a wide variance in score distribution. The extreme peaks and valleys are not evident with the mentally retarded child as they are with the child with autism.

5 1/2 YR OLD BOY: RETARDED

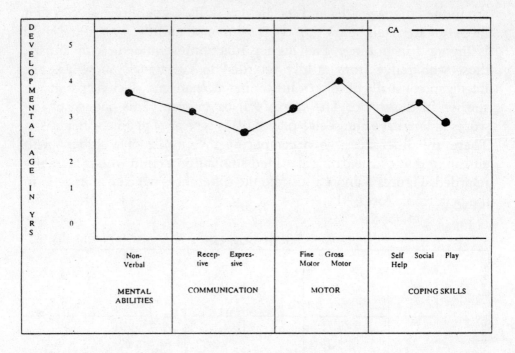

Aside from the overall uneven development, skills are not learned in the normal sequence. A child with autism may skip some developmental milestones. For example, the child may suddenly get up and walk without going through the creeping and/or crawling stages. Jumping up and down in self-stimulation may happen, but that same child may not be able to jump down from a height or jump over a rope.

DISTURBANCE OF THE SENSORY SYSTEM

The basic premise about the sensory system in people with autism is that the sensory receptors are either hypo- or hypersensitive to stimulations (Wing, 1980; Ritvo, 1978). They do not react in the same manner as others. The following are examples of disturbances with the sensory input:

Auditory

Many students with autism, at one time or another, appear to be deaf. They do not respond to sound, voices, or directions within the expected amount of response time. Sometimes this may be referred to as "selective listening" which is not the case. This seemingly willful disobedience, as mentioned previously, is not what it appears but, rather, is a delay in processing the auditory information. The processing system for many students with autism is significantly delayed which makes them appear to be deaf or selective listeners. It is a processing problem not an inability to hear or disobedience that causes this problem.

At other times these individuals may be hypersensitive or over-responsive to certain sounds such as babies crying or dogs barking. Even the anticipation of these sounds happening is enough to upset the student with autism. This may be remedied by some desensitization programs. Desensitization is a controlled, sequential exposure of the student to whatever it is (sound, activity, area) in which s/he needs to become comfortable. This takes a great deal of time and effort by a teaching staff.

Self-induced sounds such as screaming, loud hammering, or using noisy machinery/appliances can be acceptable to many of these students if they are the ones in control of the noise/sound. For example, some students with autism may overreact to another student's screams. They may begin to aggress, be self-abusive, or scream themselves when the other student begins making the loud noises. However, if the student with autism is the one who screams first, runs the vacuum, or starts the dishwasher, it generally does not upset the student. The control over the sound is important for the student with autism. The control issue comes into the picture many times with students with autism as they attempt to alleviate the confusion of their world.

Visual

Many of these students are fascinated with visual stimuli such as lights, shadows, shiny objects, reflections, spinning objects, strands of dropping pebbles, shoelaces, or recreating a favorite movement with part of their body. Hand flicking in front of the eyes is often associated with autism. One boy was observed to move his bent arm directly out from his chest and rapidly bringing it back again in succession whenever he had free time and didn't know what else to do. When asked why he moved in that manner he replied that once he rode a train, looked out the window, and that was what he saw; objects moving rapidly toward his eyes. He was recreating that pleasant sensation for himself as a form of self-stimulation.

At times, these individuals do not make any sort of eye contact with people or activities. On the other hand, they are able to complete puzzles, throw balls, or string beads accurately while seeming to stare off into space. At other times they may seem to stare through people or activities by giving intense but "sightless" eye contact. Often minute details, such as tiny specks of lint or dust on the carpet or article of clothing, are perceived by individuals with autism, yet huge obvious obstructions are "invisible" to their eyes.

Tactile

This sensation is very important, since almost everything we, as humans, do involves some touch. Eating, dressing, using teaching materials, or being around other children all involve touch. Individuals with autism do not necessarily find the same sort of touches as pleasant as the rest of the population.

Many of these people have tactile defensiveness and do not want to be touched. They will react in adverse ways to being touched even very softly. On the other hand, some people with autism may not react at all to a seemingly very painful temperature or touch. This can manifest itself in head banging, hand biting, or rubbing on hard surfaces, or pinching oneself with no apparent awareness to the pain. These behaviors are called self-abusive or self-injurious because they result in injuries the person brings on him/herself. These touches are under the control of the individual.

An increased threshold to pain is an important consideration when working with students with autism, since self-injuries may not be felt; some internal illnesses or injuries may also go unnoticed or unfelt. Earaches or severe stomachaches may go undetected and result in major physical problems.

There are also difficulties with eating and dressing which are related to textures and tactile stimulation. The great variety of food textures is disturbing to some individuals with autism. This can greatly restrict their food intake due to distinct likes or dislikes for foods. Some individuals may prefer wearing only certain clothes. These clothes may need to be a certain color, style, or feel. Loose-fitting clothes may be the preference in many cases.

Tactile stimulation involves the total being and is a difficult area in which to create desensitization programs for all aspects which can be difficult.

Olfactory/Gustatory

Students with autism may often smell or mouth/lick the many teaching materials and objects in day-to-day living. It seems almost to be an automatic response. Before they can put the peg in the board or throw the ball, it goes into their nose or mouth for a preliminary sniff or lick.

With some students functioning at a low intellectual level, licking or sniffing objects may be a form of oral stimulation. These students may actually put many different objects — leaves, pencils, paper scraps, and any other oddity found on the floor — in their mouth. Some may chew on these materials for stimulation, others may actually eat and swallow the inedible objects. A student who eats inedible objects has a disorder called pica. For the student who may be merely chewing on the objects, a substitute teething ring or appropriate chewing material may be introduced. In one instance, a student wore a teething ring at all times and was redirected to chew the teething ring when found investigating the chewable objects on the floor. In this instance the chewing of inedible objects was greatly reduced, as was the amount of time spent watching the student and removing objects from her mouth. This is not uncommon among people with autism. They require supervision and monitoring. The specific food preferences of people with autism can cause mealtimes to become major undertakings for both school and home. Some can lack in proper nutrition because of their refusal to eat a wide variety of foods. This can then become a medical problem as well.

Proprioceptive

Proprioceptive sense is the awareness one has of his/her body in space, body awareness and how to move each part of the body in useful ways. Students with autism have difficulty realizing that they are in control of their bodies, how it moves and where it moves. They may not even be aware that their feet are attached to the rest of their body. One young child with autism was reported to walk into, on and over the young baby his mother left lying on a blanket on the floor. The young boy was not aware of anything under his feet or that he was touching something. There is generally an undersensitivity to spinning on end (no dizziness), a preoccupation with spinning objects, and often continual movement such as darting, whirling and swinging when possible. Most people with autism are "earth bound" and do not realize they can get off the ground safely to ride a trike or climb a ladder. To learn many relatively simple movements, they need to be taken through the movement physically, step by step, before they are able to do the movement independently. At that point the movement may only be realized for that specific task and not generalized to other similar movements. Generalization is a very slow process, if it happens at all. Most skills learned are task specific. Throwing a basketball may be different than throwing a softball for a student with autism, or jumping down from a height may be different from jumping over a rope. Physical assistance is very important to learn the proper manner in which to perform many movement skills.

In summary, while many of the characteristics described are present in students with autism, they do not disappear with age or schooling. What can, and often does, happen is that there is a reduction of self-stimulation behaviors as more appropriate social and play skills are learned. Ways to communicate needs and wants are learned which can reduce the incidences of behavior disruptions and can provide better ways of coping with the world around them. This takes time, consistent, structured routines in the daily lives of individuals with autism, and people who understand autism as it relates to each individual specifically. With knowledgeable instructors, people with autism can learn many different skills in all areas, know success, and possibly begin to function more independently in the world.

Chapter Three

ASSESSMENT OF A STUDENT WITH AUTISM

Physical education class can be an excellent place for students with autism to enhance the areas of language and social skills which are difficult. The gym allows them the freedom to interact in leisure or structured play situations with their peers. How can an appropriate educational program be provided for students with autism? A program can be provided which emphasizes the strengths of the student in order to improve the weak areas, i.e., language and social skills, and help facilitate learning in the best possible fashion. An educational program should be directed to the total child, not exclusively classroom skills, language skills, or motor skills.

In order to get a complete picture of these students and fashion the best possible educational program, an interdisciplinary assessment which sees the total student rather than specific chunks or segments of the student is more functional in planning the school program. The interdisciplinary team may consist of a psychologist to obtain an IQ score. This would enable the team to realize the potential of the student's mental abilities. A speech/language clinician is imperative since communication is one of the weakest areas for people with autism. The clinician would be able to give invaluable information about how the student communicates, how to give the student instructions and how to understand any nonverbal communications the student may use. This information is vital for the success of the student's program at home and school. An educational consultant is another important member of the assessment team. This person can provide information regarding the type of programming the student needs within the classroom, plus information about behaviors which might occur in that setting. The fourth person on the team should be an adapted physical education specialist. Not only can the adapted physical education specialist assess gross motor skills but can also collect and share supplemental information about communication skills, behavior management strategies, teaching techniques, motivators, frustrators, play skills, interaction skills, and coping skills. This team approach can provide much valuable information about how to work with students with autism and what to expect from them in the classroom or at home.

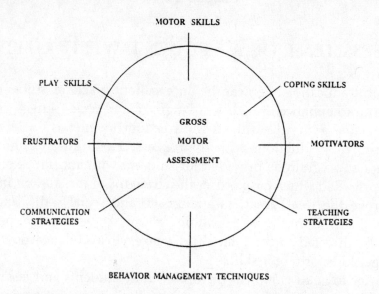

There are many areas included in a disabled student's program in which assessments are done. These assessments serve as guideposts to the development of their program. The assessment itself is not the end product, but how the assessment results are utilized are very important. Making a gross motor assessment an integral part of the educational program is essential.

GENERAL GUIDELINES UTILIZING CHARACTERISTICS FOR ASSESSING STUDENTS WITH AUTISM

When planning an assessment, it is essential to obtain information about the student to be assessed. This information should come from the student's parents, teachers and other staff who would have valuable information to share, and perhaps the student him/herself. Aside from interviews, observations of the student at school or at home can be very helpful. Videotapes are a useful tool to help facilitate viewing when actual observations are not possible.

Some general questions that the assessment team might consider to help construct the assessment itself are: What are the student's present skills in each discipline: motor, language, academic, play, social, and self-help? How does the student learn best? What are frustrators/ motivators? How can behaviors be handled? What should a program look like for the student? With questions such as these, the assessment team may be better able to accurately report the student's abilities and how to properly program for that student.

Although people with autism are different from others in a number of ways, they are also similar in some ways. It is important to note both similarities and differences when planning an assessment. There are some assessment methods which are used with the general population that can be readily used with students who are suspected of having autism. However, due to their differences, many techniques need some modification in order to use the assessment instrument with any success.

There are several general guidelines which can be very helpful when assessing these students. These guidelines are based on the characteristics discussed in the beginning of this book.

Variability

Variability among people with autism may cause the choice of one specific assessment instrument to be very difficult. Due to the wide variety among these people and lack of any standardized motor assessment that could be used and still maintain the norms, it is often more appropriate to use different segments from a variety of instruments. One instrument may assess ball skills with instructions more appropriate for a student with autism and another may assess jumping skills in a better manner. The way in which directions are given and responses accepted on standardized instruments influences the choice.

Behaviors will generally vary from student to student. Since this is true, the person doing the assessment should realize what the student is like prior to beginning an assessment. Many times the attention span of these people is very short. They are very easily distracted by activity, people, or materials in the testing environment. Some people will be fine in a large space with a great deal of equipment out, others will not. Aggression or acting-out behaviors are sometimes the only way they can express frustration or anger. For that reason it may be important for the examiner to know some basic behavior management techniques. (These will be discussed in following sections of the book.)

Depending upon the individual's tolerance to open space and large

PARENT PLANNING

CHILD:
AGE:
DOB:

PEOPLE PRESENT:

I. WHAT ARE MEG'S PROBLEMS?

1. Does Meg have other problems besides learning difficulties?
2. If so, what are they? What can you do about them?
3. What about her activity level?

II. WHAT ARE HER SKILLS?

1. What is her physical coordination ability?
2. What are her language skills?
3. What are her school skills?
4. What are her self-help skills?
5. What are her social skills?
6. What are her play skills?

III. HOW CAN WE HELP HER LEARN?

1. What kind of environment does she learn best in?
2. What motivates Meg?
3. Can she follow directions, listen? How complex—1 or 2 steps?
4. How can we help her communicate with other children in class?
5. How can you handle her fears/frustrations?
6. How can you handle her changes?
7. How can we help Meg participate in small groups?
8. How does she learn?
9. How can her behaviors be handled?
10. How can we get Meg to share control?

rooms, the examiner should determine the best place to conduct the assessment. If the assessment calls for the use of large equipment, the best place would logically be a gym or multipurpose area where equipment could be set up ahead of time. As stated, this may be a problem for some students with autism. The variability can determine many facets of the assessment from the very onset.

Qualitative Impairment of Communication

Language is one of the major areas of difficulty for people with autism. When assessing, it is imperative to know how they communicate prior to beginning the assessment. If they are to complete any aspect of the assessment, the examiner must know how to ensure that they know what they are to do. Knowing if the students are verbal or use sign language or a communication board for expressing needs is vital. Questions to answer prior to the assessment include: How much does the student comprehend? Can the student perform from a model only, a model and touch cues, or does s/he need complete physical assistance to learn how to move?

Too much language in an assessment can lead to frustration due to confusion. This frustration hinders the student's ability to perform, and therefore there may be fewer or no assessment results. By avoiding lengthy verbal directions and, instead, showing the student what is expected, there is the possibility of much more success and less frustration for both the student and the examiner. It is best to avoid talking "at" the student and using unnecessary "verbage"; instead, tell him/her precisely what s/he is to do, then assist him/her to understand and learn what those directions mean through physical assistance.

Qualitative Impairment in Interaction

In order to have the student with autism attempt assessment activities it is not so important to establish the personal (examiner/student) rapport at the beginning of the assessment. Instead, start the assessment session with motivating tasks that the student will succeed at doing. The immediate success will help keep his/her interest and enthusiasm high. People with autism do not have the understanding of personal rapport or the desire to please as others do. Throughout the session the inclusion of the successful skills will aid in keeping frustration to a minimum and a positive atmosphere during the assessment. Too many failures lead to frustration, non-compliance and unnecessary problem behaviors. A task-centered assessment with built-in success for the student rather than a people-oriented assessment will be more productive, establish a form of trust, and provide an easier time. In learning new activities most people are more willing to attempt later tasks if the beginning tasks were successful and not frustrating. Tennis, for example, would be very frustrating if on the first day everyone had to play a match. Probably very few would want to continue or return to that activity. However, if it is presented in smaller, manageable, success-oriented activities, people would be more likely to return again. This is how activities should initially be presented to the student with autism in order to have continued success.

An important point to realize when working with students with autism is that they have little desire to please anyone. People with autism generally do not do tasks to please adults. They do not have the motivation to please as others do, nor are they responsive to all adult reactions. As an examiner it is important to choose activities or toys which are motivating for the student to work for or with during the assessment period. Free time can become a motivator if it is built into the routine of the assessment. A student can be taught to work first then play, if the examiner learns what s/he wants to do, sets it aside during work time, and then guides the student to that activity or toy during play/free time. Thus, the examiner alternates work and play times. Some students may be motivated by self-stimulation; for them, toys which have the same sort of stimulating effect as their movements would be appropriate.

As well as learning the motivators, it is good to know what frustrates the students or what to avoid if at all possible. These may be things such as too much talking, unclear expectations, sudden changes, or too much physical assistance. These are very important for all staff to know while assessing a person with autism. Learning what not to do when working with a student with autism is just as important as learning what to do with that student. An assessment need not be so simple that there are no challenges. That would not be helpful, but knowing unnecessary frustrators can be very beneficial.

Many people with autism have a need for personal space and do not like being touched. This should be respected when assessing these individuals. Praise in the form of touching may actually be negative for them.

They also need to have some control over their environment, so when possible it can be good to share the control. Giving them control can be accomplished by having them help put materials away during the assessment, set up activities, as well as giving them choices such as throwing a big ball or a small ball to do a ball activity.

Predictability

Individuals with autism need structure and consistency. Preparing the student for the assessment ahead of time would benefit everyone involved. This can be done with verbal information, pictures, lists, calendars or any method which assists the student in knowing that something different will happen. Once involved in the assessment, developing a routine or structure to follow for the duration will prove helpful. The use of a "work, then play" routine is very useful and can carry over in a number of situations. Writing down what the student will do on a list which includes breaks and choices is another useful tool.

In order to determine how much structure the student in particular may require, questions may be asked. This may include: What is her/his attention span? Are there limits as to the number of repetitions or time needed? Are there physical boundaries imperative for consistency of performance? Some assessments have structure built into them by activity; most motor assessments do not. Therefore, structure should be developed. This would include the physical setup of the room and where certain activities are located within the room. Many times the more structure there is, the better the assessment will progress.

Establishing definite beginnings and endings or limits to the activities rather than having an abstract number of repetitions to do for activities is most helpful. Set limits and let the student know how many repetitions or turns s/he will have either with real objects, pictures, check marks, chips or verbal input. Giving him/her this information can alleviate some amount of stress and ease the process. For example, if s/he is to throw five balls, have five balls out to use. As s/he throws the balls, s/he can see that fewer are left as each is thrown. Once an activity is finished or the final "one more" is completed, honor that direction and reward for being finished. By respecting instructions consistently, the student can learn what to expect if "one more" is said to her/him in the assessment.

People with autism have difficulties with space and open areas. By having definite boundaries/space for activities, the student will have an easier time in the open area. During the gross motor assessment, the gym can be structured so balance activities are done in a certain area, jumping in another, and ball skills in another part of the room. Also, within each activity, boundaries or structure can be established. For example, carpet squares are an excellent and simple way to define space. The student can sit on the carpet for circle activity, stand on it to do ball skills, or jump on/over it at other times. These physical markers give the student extra clues regarding where s/he is to be and what might be expected during the activity.

Use of Sensory Stimulation

People with autism respond to sensory stimulation in ways far different from others. This should be taken into consideration when planning an assessment. The initial question might be which mode does the student use to learn: visual, tactile, auditory? As mentioned in the previous section, the responses to different sensory stimulations may be either hypo- or hyperreactive or may be delayed longer than normal in response time. This is due to confusion caused by the central nervous system problem which people with autism display.

The sensory system of a person with autism is confused and this can either be a hindrance or be used as a positive method of achieving results. Responses to different sensory input can often be used in constructive manners while assessing and programming. Reinforcement through the sensory system is an excellent method to use. Precautions must be taken as well with what input is given and how it is given.

Auditory stimulation for some people with autism should be kept to a minimum. Talking or loud noises, which are out of their control, should also be avoided. Too much talking at the student can be very disturbing, as can be loud noise. It is best to verbalize only the necessary information when giving instructions. If loud noises are unavoidable, allow the student to have some control over the noise by creating the noise or seeing what causes it. On the other hand, there may be some people with autism who do not mind being talked to or loud noises and can often be reinforced with verbal praise.

Visually, people with autism can be reinforced by their own actions such as finger flipping, spinning objects, looking in mirrors, or watching shadows. If possible, have toys available which use those movements such as windmills, tops or other infant toys.

Smelling and tasting many objects which are used for activities are other behaviors that can be used constructively. Having a favorite snack or "smelly" available for the student after each attempt at an activity can be motivating and help the student complete a task.

Touching a person with autism can be the most difficult problem for a physical education teacher, since many of them are tactilely defensive and do not respond well to touch. When assessing, it can become necessary to physically assist them to do a task initially in order for them to understand what they are to do. It may be necessary to assist the student even though s/he continually protests. With this type of student, touch may not be the appropriate method of reinforcement. By warning the student ahead of time that "I'll help you" and then giving physical assistance, some difficulties can be eliminated.

Often, gross motor activities themselves become reinforcing and no other reinforcement is necessary. All methods of reinforcement should be known ahead of time. Using the student's need for sensory stimulation is an excellent means of reinforcement for the initial assessment.

Along with each of the sensory differences should be listed the word "control." By giving them some amount of control regarding what goes on with them, they will be more likely to return to activities. For example, instead of forcing a student who does not want to do a throwing activity but has no choice about doing it, give her/him the option of throwing a big ball or little balls. Some control is then in his/her hands. Having them help set up or end activities by putting away materials is also an indication of control to them and helps them learn the differences between work and play.

By respecting their differences and using those differences in constructive manners, a great deal of hardship can be avoided. People with autism can be assessed. But in order to be successful, guidelines should be heeded. By meeting the student halfway and knowing how to deal with their special ways of learning, interacting, and communicating, the assessment process can be very successful and enjoyable for the student and examiner.

Chapter Four

MOTOR ASSESSMENT PROCEDURES

THE ROLE OF THE PHYSICAL EDUCATION/ ADAPTED PHYSICAL EDUCATION SPECIALIST

The role of the adapted physical education specialist or the physical education teacher in an assessment of a student with autism adds a unique and vital perspective. Much more than mere motor skills can be observed during a gross motor assessment. The specific objective of a gross motor assessment is to learn the strengths and weaknesses of the child in the motor domain. However, not only are gross motor skills observed but also information regarding communication skills, behavior management strategies, teaching techniques, motivators, frustrators, play skills, interaction skills, and coping skills. All of this information can be valuable for anyone who becomes involved with the education of a student with autism.

Even though the adapted physical education specialist can function and assess students with autism without input from other disciplines, it is always best to have an interdisciplinary team working to assess these students. This team approach can give all who work with these students much valuable information about how to work with them and what to expect from them in the classroom or at home. Each team member contributes to the diagnosis, assessment and programming ideas for each student to be assessed. Putting it all together is a total team effort. No one discipline can develop a comprehensive educational program for a student. Input is needed from all members of the team.

PREASSESSMENT CONSIDERATIONS

There are several items which may be helpful for the motor examiner to learn prior to the assessment which are specific to the motor area. They are:
    1. Why is the student being referred for a motor assessment?

31

This may be information to put the motor assessment in perspective with the total assessment. Is this a part of an interdisciplinary assessment with few specific motor concerns, or are there very specific motor concerns voiced by home and/or school. As the motor examiner, it is important to know specifics before beginning the assessment.

2. What are some skills the student can presently do?

This is not to take the place of the assessment but, rather, to get a starting point by learning at what age level to begin. It is good to have some idea of skill level to eliminate searching within the assessment for an appropriate beginning level.

3. Do the motor skills differ between home and school?

Many times, due to facilities, equipment, number of people, etc., students with autism display some skills at home and not at school or vice versa. This is important to learn and point out to both parents and teachers to help coordinate motor programs and to allow both groups to see all the motor skills the student does possess.

4. Which area of motor development is most difficult?

Is balance the most difficult area, or ball skills, or jumping? This information may help alleviate unnecessary frustration during the assessment process. Knowing how far to push difficult areas and which activities can be reinforcing will simplify the process.

5. What time of day will the assessment be done?

This may greatly affect the performance of the student, especially if the child is preschool age or used to taking naps in the afternoon. If it is too early or too late, the student may not perform optimally. If the motor assessment follows a long involved or difficult period/activity, the performance can also be skewed.

MOTOR ASSESSMENT SELECTION

In choosing a gross motor assessment tool, it is important to consider how functional the items on the assessment will be for the student. They need to learn skills which are practical and can be of use to them in their daily lives. These skills may be ball throwing, kicking, or catching, all of which can be used in social settings as the student grows. A great many standardized motor assessments utilize imitation of body movements, exercises, etc., which are not as likely to be used by students with autism as would ball throwing, running, jumping, and climbing, especially in the early years. Also, many times instructions for standardized testing are not understood by students with autism or are taken quite literally. This is due to the communication difficulties all students with autism encounter. For example, "stand on one foot" has caused one student to literally stand with one foot on top of the other. They often do not model from a demonstration well. Pressure to perform during standardized testing also causes difficulties. Time has little meaning for students with autism. Due to the language difficulties and problems motivating these students to perform, either a criterion-referenced assessment or a gross motor checklist would be both functional and practical. Both can be utilized while the student is involved in informal play and motor activities, as well as in structured motor tasks. In this manner, in the less formal time especially, the student has no pressure to perform and often will do many tasks better than if asked or assisted to do them. Another important aspect of these tools is that the activities are skills which can be applied to later life leisure skills, rather than some test-specific task which only measures skills specific to the assessment itself. It is important to note that the gross motor assessment for a student with autism is not so different from the assessment of a normally developing student. Differences arise from the structure and implementation of the assessment, communication techniques, behavior modification, and length of time per activity. The approach used is crucial more than the instrument.

The informal observational checklist is an important assessment tool. The examiner can obtain a feeling for the student's movement patterns through critical and sensitive observation as the student explores the environment and plays with different materials. This observation can be done in unstructured times and in more structured activity periods that involve specific tasks. In this manner, areas of both strengths and weakness can be determined. An example of a checklist is the *ISDD Gross Motor Checklist* (see Appendix).

The criterion-referenced test is very similar to an observational checklist. It is developed by determining an activity or sets of activities that the examiner wishes to observe qualitatively. The checklist is constructed to include the specific components of the skills to be observed so the examiner can systematically observe and record the movement characteristics of the student in any given moment. A criterion-referenced item makes no inference that goes beyond the movement being observed. Criterion-referenced items can be constructed for any skill, so it is flexible and a useful tool. An example of a criterion-referenced test is the

Institute for the Study of Developmental Disabilities Gross Motor Assessment (see Appendix).

Students with autism can be assessed successfully using either of these instruments. The reason these instruments are successful is that they can be more informal and unstructured observations of the student rather than a formalized type of assessment. As mentioned, the student may not feel threatened or under pressure to do well in these types of assessments. The more relaxed the student can be, the more apt s/he may be to attempt different activities. Success can be built into these types of situations as a reinforcement. Simple observation of the students at play can tell the examiner a great deal without actually "testing."

In working with students with autism, the author has used both of the above instruments while participating in interdisciplinary assessments. The results from the checklist and/or the criterion-referenced checklist most consistently coincide with small gross motor sections on the Vineland Adaptive Behavior Scales (an interview with the parents and teachers of the student) and the PEP (Psychoeducational Profile) which was specifically designed for students with autism. These instruments appear complete enough to cover the gross motor skill needs of students with autism.

STRUCTURE OF THE ASSESSMENT

The structure of the motor assessment does not need to be totally formal. It is often best if all of the specific areas to be used for activities are established prior to the actual assessment. All materials should be readily available for the examiner. Balance activities could be set up in one area of the room and ball activities in another. This structure helps to give order to a somewhat unstructured, cluttered open area which might be difficult for a student with autism to handle.

Generally, an assessment can be completed in an hour. Less time is required if the student is so severely retarded or behaviors are so interfering that it may be difficult to continue for that amount of time. For most students with autism, an hour is a good session and can be done due to the fact that most of them have fairly intact motor skills and they seem to enjoy a variety of these activities.

FREE TIME OBSERVATIONS

Since these students display a variety of ability, understanding, interests, etc., some adaptations to the assessment procedures are necessary, especially for the more severely retarded students with autism. Rather than beginning the assessment immediately, it is very beneficial to allow the student time to explore the room and equipment which will be used. By giving the student free time to explore without any adult interferences, it is possible to notice other aspects of the student. What might be observed during this time is very helpful in diagnosis and programming. The following are aspects of the student, other than gross motor, which can be observed and noted during this free time span.

1. How does the student adapt to large open spaces? This is often difficult for students with autism due to lack of boundaries or controlling influences.

2. What equipment does the student choose to play with on her/his own? These can be used as motivators, reinforcers or success-oriented activities to utilize when the student becomes frustrated.

3. What are potential frustrators? Along with the above-mentioned motivators, activities or toys which do not appeal to the child can be observed and then avoided during the assessment, unless absolutely necessary for the assessment procedure.

4. How does the student communicate? This is very important information which can be contributed to any team working with students with autism. Many times gross motor activities are very motivating for these students and they indicate the desire for more in a number of ways. These methods can often be shaped into functional communication techniques such as signing or the use of a communication board, or single word requests.

5. Does the student display any type of problem-solving skills? This can be seen as the student tries to get a ball which is out of reach or climbs over/under obstacles, or attempts to communicate these needs to someone. This is an indication of learning abilities that are important when developing the student's educational program.

6. What are the student's play/social skills independently or with others? Observing play/social skills is an essential part of an interdisciplinary assessment. Students with autism do not generally use pretend play but, rather, play in very ritualistic manners. Any interaction can

also be noted whether it is to play or merely gain a desired object or help. All play or interaction attempts are important pieces of the puzzle.

7. Movement skills which are the core of the motor assessment can be observeed while the student is not pressured to perform. Often the child will be more comfortable in free time movement rather than in a more structured setting.

This observation time is essential and important information for all involved in working with the student with autism.

ASSESSMENT FORMULA

OBSERVATION PERIOD
(5–7 MIN)

—COPING WITH SPACE
—CHOICE OF EQUIPMENT
—POSSIBLE MOTIVATORS/FRUSTRATORS
—HOW CHILD COMMUNICATES
—PROBLEM SOLVING THROUGHOUT ROOM
—HOW CHILD PLAYS ALONE/INTERACTS
—MOVEMENT SKILLS

TECHNIQUES FOR STRUCTURED ACTIVITIES

Once the initial observation is over, the more structured assessment can take place. The assessment will include a variety of skills which the student may have done in free time and other skills not yet attempted. Normal assessment procedures cannot often be followed when working with a student with autism. The examiner needs to ensure that the child understands what is expected per activity in order to determine how a best performance looks.

A way to help this understanding is to structure the room so there are specific areas for each activity. The room should be arranged ahead of time whenever possible. For example, in one corner of the room have all the balance and jumping activities set up, possibly in an obstacle course. In another area have targets on the wall for ball-tossing games and assessment.

The "Three-Step Approach" to having a student initiate a movement is:

1) State the direction and point toward the activity . . . wait
2) State the direction and model the movement . . . wait
3) State the direction and physically assist to complete the task

Once the student is involved in the activity, have him/her repeat it three times whenever possible. The first time total assistance may be necessary due to the student's inability to understand what is being requested. On the second attempt give minimal assistance and the third time allow the student to be independent. If the student can be independent sooner, allow that to happen. Independence in movement and skills is one of the ultimate goals for these children. This process can be done with all motor skills on the assessment. There are times when the actual assessment activities are completed and the student appears not to be able to do skills, but then the student will attempt the skills on his/her own in free time between activities. Once they understand what is expected of them and know how to move, they often take the initiative to do the skills.

STRUCTURED ACTIVITIES THREE STEP APPROACH
1. STATE DIRECTION AND POINT TOWARD ACTIVITY . . . WAIT
2. STATE DIRECTION AND MODEL THE MOVEMENT . . . WAIT
3. STATE DIRECTION AND PHYSICALLY ASSIST
ONCE INVOLVED IN THE ACTIVITY, REPEAT THE TASK THREE TIMES
1. FIRST TIME GIVE TOTAL PHYSICAL ASSISTANCE (IF NEEDED)
2. SECOND TIME REDUCE PHYSICAL ASSISTANCE
3. THIRD TIME ALLOW INDEPENDENCE
BY LEARNING HOW TO DO THE SKILL, THE CHILD SHOULD BE ABLE
TO DO THE SKILL INDEPENDENTLY BY THE THIRD TIME THROUGH.

Throughout the assessment, the use of the various motivators/reinforcers observed during the initial few minutes is useful. The contingency method of "First work, then play" is a simple strategy. The wording can change, "First climb ladder, then bubbles," to suit the activity. Another technique for a more difficult student is to tell him/her what to do and if s/he refuses tell him/her, "I'll help you throw the ball: 1-2-3 . . ." and then physically assist to the task. Whatever strategy is chosen, it should be used consistently by all working with the student in order for it to have any effect on the student.

If, on the other hand, a student seems receptive to more repetitions of a certain skill and willing to try variations of the skill, stay with it for awhile. This can give valuable information not only about motor skills but also about how long the student can stay with a task that is pleasurable. Care must be taken to prevent constant perseveration of the activity, but rather that the student do the activity when requested and be willing to stop at any given time.

Praise and reinforcement throughout the assessment is a motivator for some students (while it remains unmotivating to others) and they will be encouraged. In all cases, it is good to be as positive as possible and encourage the student throughout the assessment.

Chapter Five

INTERPRETATION AND
REPORTING ASSESSMENT FINDINGS

UNEVEN DEVELOPMENT

The results of an interdisciplinary assessment are shared with the entire team. Each team member's input can greatly contribute to the total picture of the child. At the information-sharing meeting a developmental profile can be constructed using the findings from each discipline and assessment instrument. An example of a profile shown here is the typical pattern found in people with autism. The uneven rate of development which was discussed in the overview is illustrated:

5 1/2 YR OLD BOY: AUTISM

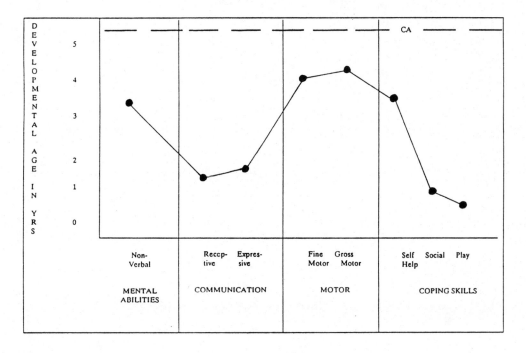

The lowest areas will always be in the language, social, and play categories.

When the team discusses the results, the (adapted) physical education teacher will be able to report the gross motor score. Since each area can develop unevenly, a solid point can be placed on the profile where most skills cluster and skills higher or lower may be indicated by a wavy line. The range of skills can then be seen at a glance. Not only can the A.P.E. teacher report the motor scores but also can contribute to the communication section and to the "Next Step" teaching strategies or educational program ideas.

The assessment serves as a guidepost for the development of the student's program. It is important that the results be treated in a useful and practical manner. The interdisciplinary team's job does not stop once the results are charted. Their continued sharing of how they answered the assessment planning questions about how the student learns, behaviors to control, how to get the student to work in their disciplines, how to communicate, what motivates/frustrates the student, how the student plays, and how the student responds to different behavior management strategies are vital for the assessment to be a totally useful process.

The ideas generated at the information-sharing staffing after the assessment can be incorporated into the interdisciplinary report as general recommendations. As each team member assessed the student, the examiner was looking for answers to the preassessment questions as well as information specific to their respected areas. Since each member has information to share which affects the student's ability to work, the information is shared and compiled into the recommendations that can be used by all disciplines. As the following example shows, the general recommendations are generic and do apply to all areas. They can then be incorporated into a report that also includes discipline-specific information as well. A sample of this interdisciplinary brainstorming follows:

1. How does Meg learn?

    A. Use of routine during the day
    B. Successful activities
    C. Show her what to do, clear expectations
    D. Use short, simple, direct language
    E. Be firm when necessary, avoid verbal coaxing
    F. Let her have some control
    G. Make tasks fun

    H. For learned tasks, work at a table

    I. For new work, work in a variety of places

2. What is motivating?

    A. Adult attention, praise, free time

3. What is frustrating?

    A. Too much table work

    B. Too much physical assistance

4. How can we get Meg to be independent and/or work in a group?

    A. Build it into her routine

    B. Start with things she can do

    C. Short sessions

    D. Adult direction

    E. Begin with something she likes

5. What should Meg's program be?

    A. Small classroom ratio

    B. Structured

    C. Social, verbal peers

6. How can her behaviors be handled?

    A. Understand her behaviors and why they occur

    B. Make sure she understands what she is to do

    C. Make sure she can do "it."

    D. Ignore and redirect

    E. Tell her what to do, not what not to do

    F. Limit language

    G. Don't let her tantrums get her out of work

REPORT FORMAT

The gross motor report should be written clearly, simply, practically as a whole and per discipline. It is important to include both the strengths and weaknesses the student displayed without dwelling on either. It is already apparent that these children have difficulties in skill development; for that reason it might be highly beneficial to point out more constructive results from the assessment. In other words, report the problems, but then offer suggestions to help improve the quality of the movements. By conveying how the program can help rather than how hopeless the situation might be, a more positive use of the assessment is demonstrated. This does not mean mislead parents or other school personnel with glorified results, but be honest and point out possible "can do" skill builders to keep enthusiasm and interest high.

When writing gross motor recommendations keep in mind how useful and functional they are for the student and how easily they can be implemented by the parents and school. The recommendations which are included in the report most generally can form the backbone of the IEP and programming which are used by the school. The more functional the assessment report is, the more useful it will be to those who read it.

Chapter Six

PROGRAMMING ADAPTED PHYSICAL EDUCATION

USING THE REPORT FOR THE IEP

Programming is related very closely to the assessment results. Once the assessment report is written and recommendations generated, the next step is an IEP (individualized education plan) meeting. The (adapted) physical education teacher should be a part of that meeting.

According to PL 94-142 physical education is included within the "special education" and is "to be specifically designed instruction at no cost to parents or guardians to meet the unique needs of the handicapped child" (Education for All Handicapped Children Act 1975, Sec. 4-16). In order to ensure this service to the student, specific goals and objectives should be included on each student's IEP. The motor section should incorporate the assessment results and recommendations.

The IEP goals and objectives for the gross motor section, as well as the other areas, do not need to be complicated but should allow for some amount of challenge and success. Realistic, functional goals and objectives are most important to keep in mind when writing the IEP. Not only will the (adapted) physical education teacher prepare the motor objectives but also have input into the general behavioral objectives which are skills not specific to any discipline but have an effect on the student as a whole such as those mentioned in the general recommendations.

The following are samples of several gross motor recommendations which have been used with students with autism.

- Individualized adapted physical education which stresses basic gross motor skills and simple interactive game skills.
- Throwing or kicking balls to targets or adults
- Riding a tricycle for 20 feet independently
- Jumping down from various heights independently
- Participation in circle games with peers
- Complete the AAHPERD Physical Fitness Tests

- Participation in recess-type activities such as hopscotch, jump rope or four-square
- Swim the length of the pool with adult assistance
- Learn the names of the bases in baseball
- Independently complete a circuit training course of physical fitness exercises
- Ride a bicycle 50 yards independently

FROM IEP TO LESSON PLAN

Lesson plans can be an offshoot of the IEP if they are written properly. Students with autism need to have consistent structured routines which can be built into lessons. These plans can be divided into the general motor areas as is the assessment—locomotor, jumping, and ball skills and play equipment. Within these areas a variety of activities can be included which emphasize the student's motoric needs.

All students with autism need structure within their lessons, especially initially. The routine helps children learn task expectations, success, and increase their willingness to comply. Due to the short attention span of the students, a great deal and variety of skills are included. In this manner, the teacher is not at a loss for an activity that needs to be developed or improved. Not all of the activities are accomplished in any one lesson, but they are there to reduce boredom, frustration, and problems for both teacher and student. By establishing a consistent routine with a variety of activities, the student can be assured of having a success-oriented adapted physical education class. The more success they have, the more confidence they acquire in their ability to perform and are more willing to persevere.

Throughout the lesson it is important to remember that students with autism learn best through routine, structure, and consistency. Repetition of the same lesson plan will enable the student to learn more readily. The teacher should be as positive as possible during the lesson, giving encouragement every step of the way. By ensuring successes, the student will have good and positive feelings regarding the gross motor skills in the lesson. The success of the student in gross motor skills can greatly enhance the self-concept which may overflow into other areas. Therefore, it is extremely important to help the student succeed and have as positive an outlook as possible.

CLASS STRUCTURE

Low Functioning Students With Autism

The lower functioning students with autism, those who are also moderately to severely retarded, will need one-to-one individualized adapted physical education. These students have very poor proprioceptive (body awareness) skills and are not aware of what their bodies can do or how their bodies move. They will need a great deal of physical assistance to put them through many of the activities. In working with lower functioning students with autism, the approach that was used for the assessment, "The Three-Step Approach," can be followed. A consistent structured routine should be established and a variety of activities should be included within the program due to the very short attention span of most of these students. The more varied and the more success-oriented those activities can be, the more willing the student will be to participate in the program. The program itself should include areas of all basic gross motor skills: balance, locomotor, body projection, ball skills, and play skills. They need to be shown how to do the activities and cannot be expected to do the activities as soon as they walk into the gross motor area. They do not have the ability or awareness of what is going on around them and do not learn how to do activities as the other students do from watching or experimenting. They need to be helped a great deal at first.

As these students progress and are involved in the daily routine which is consistent and structured, less physical assistance will be needed and their independence will grow. One of the ultimate goals of the motor program, as well as the total program, is that the student learn to function without adult assistance being necessary. The routine helps to speed up that process.

High Functioning Students With Autism

Higher functioning students with autism, students who are mildly mentally retarded to average or above average intelligence, will also need some initial physical assistance. These children may have the movements down but will be very awkward and somewhat unsure of the movements. Guidance through the movements can improve their quality so they can better fit into game situations. This is necessary to help them achieve a certain level of success. These students also need work on some of the basic gross motor skills in order to have success when integrated into other classes. They will be more likely to play a game of soccer, for example, or a game of kickball than will the moderately mentally retarded student with autism. However, lower functioning students can also learn those skills, but they will need almost complete adult assistance to have successful participation. The higher functioning students will not require as much adult assistance to participate successfully.

LEAST RESTRICTIVE ENVIRONMENT OPTIONS

All students should have the opportunity to be in a least restrictive environment (LRE) if at all possible. In some instances this may mean that the higher functioning students with autism will not be in an adapted physical education class all of the time but will be integrated into regular physical education classes. Care should be taken when this is done to ensure that the activities are within the physical and mental realm of the student. Games and activities that require a very fast pace for an extended period of time such as basketball may not be too wise a choice for some students. This is an individual matter and should be treated as such.

Students who are higher functioning may be placed in a regular physical education class. They will possibly require some initial orientation to the rules in the class or an adult to go with them for a few days until they can follow routine and understand the games that are being played. Sometimes, the games that are played in class can be practiced in the adapted physical education class. All students should have the opportunity to be with sociable, verbal peers and physical education class is an excellent place for that to take place. There is always a great deal of socialization and communication that goes on during class and the student with autism can build upon those skills during the class time naturally. Physical education class builds the student's social skills, communication skills, as well as the student's self-concept, body awareness and physical skills. While the student's skills are improving, the teacher can work with behavior management strategies that are needed and utilize different teaching techniques that can help the student improve and achieve.

Another way to allow students with autism to integrate with normally developing students is to bring the normally developing students into an adapted physical education class to act as buddies or models. This may be a better method for the lower functioning students. By bringing students into the adapted class, the students with autism do not have the anxieties that may be created by going to a new room/gym and being with so many new students. This also allows the normally developing students an opportunity to get to know the students with autism and feel more comfortable with them. Developing a buddy system is an excellent way to free the teacher and build socialization and communication skills and, at the same time, improve motor skills.

Many times people decide that integrating the students with autism is the best possible solution for them without considering the tasks and activities the student has to do. Any student when placed in a situation where the task is too difficult or who has no success will increase his/her negative behaviors and refusal behaviors. These students will not have the desire to return to that situation. If the student with autism is forced to attend a physical education class in which the pace is too fast or the activities are above his/her physical or mental abilities, negative behaviors will increase and the desire to go back will decrease as well. There will need to be more effort by the teacher to control the student and keep the student involved. When integrating a student into a least restrictive environment it should be done when the activities are appropriate. A basketball game may not be the best possible way of integrating a student with autism. It is not that they shouldn't play basketball, but it may be very frustrating for the student. They may be able to be included in aerobics, volleyball, swimming, badminton, kickball or softball, but very fast-paced games are not the best initial point to integrate. At some point, the high functioning students should be included, but the teacher needs to take care and watch for an increase in frustration and be sure there is some activity that is very successful and reinforcing for the student to do when s/he is taken from the game.

LRE is an important aspect of the student's education, but it should include an appropriate placement. Monitoring the activities through careful observation is a very important aspect of the teacher's job. Being sure that the student with autism does not become frustrated or lose the desire to participate and communicate with peers is essential. The class should be made as safe and successful for that student as possible.

CIRCUIT TRAINING

As well as working on basic gross motor skills such as catching, kicking, throwing, or jumping, youth with autism need programs which include physical fitness. A great many of them can become rather lethargic and do not know how to become involved in an activity; or can become highly active in an inappropriate, hyperactive fashion. This lack or abundance of energy should be channeled into an appropriate mode of activity. An individualized fitness program designed per student would be one way to involve the students in constructive activities.

There are a great many fitness programs on the market today, but each person needs one designed specifically to meet his/her physical needs and limitations. A routine can be established which can be followed daily, or every other day which would be valuable to the total person, physically, mentally, and socially. As it becomes part of each person's day the benefits would grow. Since students with autism require some consistent structure for activities, a set "circuit training" pattern can be developed to meet the needs and exercise the entire body. The circuit can include jogging, walking, swimming, exercise bike riding, weight training, aerobics, and simple exercises. As the circuit becomes part of the daily routine, increases in repetitions or weights can be done.

Initially, each student will need some individualized assistance to understand what is to be done during the circuit time. Demonstration or physical assistance may have to be employed to ensure success and understanding of each activity. Independence in doing the circuit is one of the ultimate goals of developing a circuit training program. Verbal direction may be necessary to get the student started, but once into the established routine, it is hoped that only verbal cues would be necessary to guide the student through his/her routine. For some students the use of a written chart telling of the exercises and number is helpful. Another possibility is the use of pictures of the exercise or activity and a number for repetitions. In most instances having the necessary equipment out at its respective station so the student can see all that is available to be done is one of the best methods of helping the student grasp the routine. Each student will need an individualized approach to increase understanding and awareness of the activities to be done.

One program which is specifically designed for special populations comes from the AAHPERD–Kennedy Foundation and is a Special Fitness Test which includes seven categories: flexed arm hang, sit-ups, shuttle run, standing broad jump, 50-yard dash, softball throw, and 300-yard run-walk. These activities can all be done by students with autism.

The best way to establish a proper circuit for youth with autism is to assess their abilities and needs, then plan their circuit training program. Abilities do not mean only physical, but communication for understanding directions and behavioral needs as well. The instructor needs to establish the communication, design the gym or available space so activities are consistently in one place, and provide the guidance each student requires. As the routine becomes part of the day, the instructor's job is one of cues and redirection rather than demonstration or assistance.

The following are samples of lessons/activities that have been used successfully with different students with autism.

I. Mike is a highly verbal student and can read. A point system has been designed by the interdisciplinary team working with Mike for behavior control. The point system is incorporated into all of Mike's lessons. This activity sheet is given to Mike when he comes into the gross motor room. He is then given only reminders to stay on task. The limits or repetitions have been changed regularly and he is warned ahead of time that the numbers would be changing to challenge him.

MIKE'S P.E. ACTIVITIES

Following the rules of:

1. Starting on time	2
2. Completing each task	2
3. Doing each task well	2
4. Resting short periods	2
5. Finishing on time	2

Mike will earn 10 points doing the following:

1. Sit-ups _____
2. Leg lifts _____
3. Standing broad jump _____ (4 times)
4. Shuttle run _____ sec. (3 times)
5. Flexed arm hang _____
6. Toe touches _____
7. Push-ups _____
8. Arm circles _____
9. Play catch _____
10. Shoot baskets — make _____

II. Sara worked for stickers as a reinforcer; if she completed a task she received a sticker which she placed on her chart. Sara kept her charts. She worked best if the instructor participated rather than acted as a "cue giver." She was also working on playground/recess activities to prepare her for the public school setting to which she would return.

SARA'S A.P.E. WORK   STICKERS

1. Sit-ups
2. Toe touches
3. Arm circles
4. Shuttle run
5. Long Jump
6. Higher and lower
7. Hopscotch
8. 4-square
9. 50-yard dash
10. Surprise activity

III. David had no written chart but relied on the organization and placement of activities in the gym. He initially needed a great deal of verbal direction/demonstration to perform activities in proper manner but soon became independent. Ten activities were always out and available for him to do, and he knew he had to complete them all properly before he could have free time. David had the freedom to choose the order of the activities. The cues given to David were verbal as to repetitions and asking "What's next today" and visual cards with a picture and the word of the activity depicted. He became very independent in his routine which included physical fitness skills, most especially exercises.

The three samples included activities other than strictly physical fitness; those students needed those skills within their routine also. The following are possible suggestions for a "circuit training" physical fitness program including stretching, exercises, weights, and some aerobic type of exercise.

Establish within the gym or activity room the station area: sit-ups done on mats, weight lifting at the weight bench, etc. Written signs saying STATION 1, STATION 2, etc. plus the activity can be helpful. Assist each student through his/her routine until some degree of independence has been established, then fade guidance and instructions.

Utilize pictures, simple written instructions or numbers at each station to help the student's learning of the routine.

Possible Stations:

1. Stretching—warm-ups of entire body
2. Sit-ups
3. Toe touches   all done on a mat
4. arm circles   (1–4)
5. squats
6. curls
7. bench press
8. toe raise   weight bench—have
9. triceps lift   picture and number of
10. dumbbell fly   repetitions listed
11. leg lift   5–12)
12. arm rowing
13. exercise bike/jogging/aerobic workout

These all can be varied as needed. A timer used when riding the exercise bike helps limit the length of time for the student. Five minutes is a good starting time.

Aerobic exercise can be developed to go along with the songs the students enjoy. Simple exercises or movements incorporated with the music is aerobic exercise. Jogging can be done inside or outside. Establish a clearly marked path for the students to follow. Initial assistance may be needed to help the students understand how to use the path. Start with short distances and gradually increase distance or time for each student.

Some sample IEP objectives may read:

_____ will increase jogging distance to one mile
_____ will increase weight-lifting repetitions by 3
_____ will ride the exercise bike 10 minutes
_____ will complete circuit training program with minimal redirection

This form of adapted physical education can be used with both high and low functioning students with autism. The amount of independence, repetitions and time duration will vary accordingly. This is a good method to utilize when the teacher has a group of students of varying skills.

Chapter Seven

TEACHING STRATEGIES

When instructing a student with autism in physical education or any discipline, there are some simple, basic guidelines to remember. These can be applied in the gym, classroom, on a bus, or at home—anywhere the person has to go. The major areas are communication, behavior and skill acquisition.

COMMUNICATION

Communication is a major concern with students with autism, which can be a cause of difficulties with learning and, also, with behavior. Emphasis on appropriate communication throughout the day by all staff should be a vital part of the student's program. Once the best means of communication has been determined (signing, communication board), the entire staff must be consistent in using it. The directions which are given must be realistic for the student. When stated, the directions should be concrete, short phrases paired with gestures, signs or the communication board/card. Any extra language or talking should be eliminated when giving directions, especially when initially expecting a student to follow the direction. S/he needs to learn to listen to the verbalization and respond appropriately; any extra language may cause confusion. Telling the students what they are to do rather than what not to do also helps them to pair a direction with a desired response/action. Another way of helping the student learn meanings of directions is to use the same phrases across disciplines throughout the day, i.e., "Show me _____," "Touch _____," "One more time," "Come sit," or "First work, then _____." When using phrases, talk at a slower pace and avoid too many directions at once. It is best to pause between directions to give the student a chance to process the words.

Eliciting communication from these students is more difficult; they need to have a reason to communicate before they attempt to "reach out." It is up to the teacher to set up situations which encourage communication.

Setting up situations to encourage communication such as keeping a desired food or toy out of reach or putting desired objects in a tightly closed container are methods which can be attempted. It is important to set up these situations, since people with autism do not readily indicate wants or needs. Once they are interested in communicating their wants/needs, every attempt to communicate must be rewarded immediately. Reward the child when they are looking at a desired object, reaching, touching your hand which is on the object, gesturing, vocalizations, words, signs, and/or pointing to the objects. Success in communicating is very important for the students to achieve. Initially physical assist to provide success, eliminate frustration and provide a model. As they learn how to communicate and get results, more skills can be shaped. The use of motivating activities is often the best means to begin to elicit communication. It is important to be consistent in the expectations and reinforcements.

The interaction time is there in leisure situations with their peers and communication opportunities arise. Many times for the lower functioning students with autism, the desire for "more" of a favorite activity/movement becomes very apparent and the student can be shaped to communicate "more" in some appropriate functional fashion such as signing, a communication board, or making the sound of "more." This can be shaped each time the teacher does the activity. Do the activity, stop the activity and ask the student, "What do you want?" and then watch for the student's method of communicating.

Many times an activity can become a student's favorite and s/he will indicate the desire for "more" in some fashion. The communication of "more" can be shaped to an appropriate and functional mode each time this activity is desired. Also, shaping interaction with other students can be facilitated in class by instructing models with techniques about teaching what to say and do in order to get the student with autism to complete activities in class time.

Gestures need to be very concrete and consistent with all people who work with these students. Gestures such as "sit down" and patting a chair or "come here" are fairly universal and more readily understood by most students. Communication must be concrete and not subtle in order to get through to the person with autism.

BEHAVIOR MANAGEMENT

Many people with autism display acting-out behaviors or self-stimulation which interferes with learning. There are methods of behavior management and organization which can help reduce or eliminate interfering behaviors.

Organization of the physical environment and the student's day is one method to help control behaviors. Establish a motor routine which is consistent and structured for the student. As this becomes learned and the student knows what is first in the routine, next, etc., his/her anxiety or unwillingness to work should reduce. A way to help some students learn their routine is through the use of a schedule book. This is a personal book with drawings or pictures on note cards bound together which represent the day's events—i.e., motor room pictures for motor time, record player picture for music, etc. This can enhance learning and may also be used by the student to indicate wants.

Contingencies, using the "First work, then (play)," should also be used across settings. Many times the students will initially need physical assistance to complete a direction and learn expectations. However, as the student learns the contingencies and expectations, the physical assistance should fade and gradual independence should emerge when given the direction using the chosen communication system for that student.

Besides the consistent structured routine, it also helps to have clear boundaries or exact places to sit, stand, etc. The use of carpet squares or small chairs for their place gives them a concrete place to be when not always engaged in an activity. The use of the phrase "out of bounds" when they get into something they shouldn't is more generic and positive than a flat "no," and it can be used very broadly indicating places, objects, and activities.

As stated earlier when giving directions, be sure the expectations are realistic and clearly, but simply, stated. Telling the student what to do and ignoring inappropriate behavior and redirecting to the appropriate behavior is essential, i.e., "pick up crayons," rather than, "If you don't pick up, you can't go to gym." Often it is best to state the directions three times, with time between each direction, and then physically assist through the activity. Physical assistance helps the child understand the expectations; as s/he learns, less physical assistance will be necessary. Giving the students warnings of what is next also helps; for example, as the students come to a task, tell him/her, "You'll walk the balance beam three times, then finished." As s/he finishes each crossing remind the student, "Two/one more, then finished." Having definite beginnings and endings to tasks helps set expectations for them and reduces anxiety about how long or how many. By having all the balls to throw together or placing a line on the pages of a paper for letter writing (c _ _ _ _) gives them some indication of when they will be finished and what they have to do. The more ordered and structured their day, the better the behavior.

Ideally, each student should have a behavior plan listing behaviors to be increased or decreased and what the interventions for each behavior will be (see Appendix for behavior plan). This can help staff to be consistent in dealing with outbursts or disruptive behaviors. Also, on the chart/plan it is good to list motivators and reinforcers. Often, reinforcers are necessary in helping the student manage their behavior. Keep a list, but be aware that reinforcers can change often. Use a reinforcer initially even after one response; then lengthen the time or number of activities between reinforcers.

Objects which the students attaches to may be used as reinforcers during work time, but s/he may need it unconditionally during free time. Along with object attachment, self-stimulation may initially be used as a reinforcer. Some students may like to use their fingers to flick in front of their face as a stimulation; control this while working by holding one hand down and using the other to work or both to work. When the activity is completed, allow the self-stimulation. Those behaviors usually decrease when play and communication skills increase. Redirecting the student to play appropriately is often necessary. Unless the behaviors are self-injurious, there may need to be some time when it is okay to engage in self-stimulation. Providing OK places for the student is a way to differentiate work and play areas/times.

For behaviors which do require negative reinforcement, use a "quick sit." For example, if a student is physically aggressive, tell him/her, "The rule is no hurting" and help him/her to "sit (directly on the floor) then play game." Give no attention until the student is calm, then redirect him/her to "play game." If the behavior is uncontrollable, the student may need to "sit out," which is being removed from group attention for a specified time in a specific area. State the rule and have the student sit for two or three minutes or until calm. Then redirect the student back to the activity.

In order to keep a record of problem behaviors and what interventions work, it would be beneficial for the staff to keep some simple data or chart behaviors. Then the sharing of that information at a staffing to discuss possible alternatives would be valuable to keep consistency in the program.

It may be the case when a student is "bad" that those giving instructions need to rethink and listen critically to what they have said to the student and be sure that the instructions were clear and that they were understood. If understanding is made easier for these students through the use of consistent, structured routines and language that is concrete and concise, behavior problems can sometimes be avoided.

METHODS

Students with autism do not learn how to play by merely observing others playing; they need to be shown and physically assisted through the motions of whatever the play might be, rolling a ball to a partner or riding a trike. Structured play sessions are needed for students with autism to learn how to occupy their time appropriately.

Due to the unpredictability of peers, teachers must help both the student with autism and their schoolmates with their interactions. Teaching/modeling appropriate interactions skills should be a high priority, since this is one of the weakest areas of development for people with autism. Helping them learn turn taking, movements for simple games or playground skills will be necessary in the student's school day. Schoolmates can be taught how to give instructions in simple ways and to wait for the student with autism to respond since s/he may be a bit slower than usual.

In school, consistency and routine can be followed by having the same activities take place at the same time each day. Within activities, a routine should also be as consistent as possible. For example, in the motor room have the student do the activity routine in the same manner daily, use the same directions per activity, and be consistent with expectations. One other way to help the student cope with change or transition from one activity to another is to give the student some warning of what will happen or be expected. This can be done in a number of ways: verbally, with checklists, with pictures, drawings, or with some physical indication of change. The warnings should be given well enough in advance to allow the student time to process all of the information. Many times within lessons telling the student, "one more time, then play" etc. gives the student an indication of the expectations.

Many times unexpected changes do occur and cannot always be explained ahead of time, such as fire drills. For those types of situations some solutions are to practice ahead of time what to do when the fire alarm goes off. That is a very functional skill for anyone to learn and it could become part of a lesson for the students. If the students have some idea of what to do when strange sounds occur, it can reduce the anxiety and alleviate problem behaviors. Another possible solution to the problems which can take place is to get the student back into activities within the routine which are safe and successful. Rather than trying to comfort or control the behavior with lengthy explanations which will not be understood, get the student back into the normal routine of the day to help him/her see that all is right and the day will go on as usual.

When teaching students with autism, it should not be assumed that all underlying skills are learned or that they should be learned. It is not necessarily important to break a skill down into its component parts if the student is already doing the task in its entirety. For example, if a student is reading whole words, it may cause more problems trying to get the student to learn the ABC's rather than presenting new whole words. Help the student progress from his/her present level of functioning to move forward in learning.

Chapter Eight

SUMMARY

Every individual has the right to an education as written in PL 94-142. Based on the information written herein, certain assumptions can be made regarding the education of a person with autism. Each person has unique abilities which must be recognized by teachers in order to promote learning. Guidelines and suggestions have been generated and set forth for educators' use in planning their teaching strategies. Many of the strategies are already employed by teachers and would not be unique to the educational practices for people with autism.

When teaching, it is best to have a plan (daily, weekly, or monthly) to help set the range of activities to be explored. Maintaining a consistent, structured routine assists students in becoming familiar with expectations behaviorally, as well as educationally. This is especially true of people with autism. Use of clear, concise language facilitates ease of learning for students with autism and is a good general practice for instruction of all students. Socialization is inherent in most educational practices through the group process of games, squads, reading groups, and basic classroom time. This is a necessary part of education for all people, not a specialized skill for people with autism.

There are different learning styles, different needs, different abilities among people with autism, just as there are among the population in general. People with autism merely make those differences more or (at times) less noticeable. Teachers need to adjust to these differences. Some may argue that is too mammoth a task for a teacher to undertake; in a few instances that may be true. However, as teachers it is our responsibility to face the differences head on and develop strategies for teaching and promoting learning. This is the challenge. Interdisciplinary approaches increase the flow of ideas and keep morale up while maximizing the students' level of learning.

APPENDICES

ISDD GROSS MOTOR CHECKLIST, ASSESSMENTS, AND REPORTS

ISDD GROSS MOTOR CHECKLIST

Name: _____ Age: _____ Date: _____

Key to Abilities

I — Independent   T — Total Assistance   U — Unable to do

M — Minimal Assistance   R — Refused   D — Did not attempt

— CHECK the appropriate skill performance and indicate ability level using the Key to abilities.

ACTIVITIES	NORMS	COMMENTS
Static Balance Skills		
STAND		
. . . pulls self onto knees		
. . . stand 5 seconds — no support	0–12 months	
. . . stand alone well		
. . . kneels alone		
. . . stand on one foot w/help	13–24 months	
. . . move from sit to stand		
. . . stand or tiptoe — demonstrated with assistance		
. . . balance on one foot one second	25–36 months	
& 5 seconds with assistance		
. . . balance on tiptoes (to reach)		
. . . balance on one foot (5 secs.) 2 of 3 attempts	37–48 months	
. . . balance skillfully on toes to run		
. . . balance on one foot 10 seconds 2 of 3 attempts	49–60 months	
. . . balance on tiptoes 10		

ACTIVITIES	NORMS	COMMENTS
seconds with hands on hips 1 of 3 attempts		
... stand on one foot 10 seconds, eyes closed	61–72 months	
SIT—SQUAT		
... sit—slight support/no support	0–12 months	
... lowers self from stand to sit		
... seats self in small chair		
... squats in play	13–24 months	
... squats and returns to stand		
WALK		
... creep (F)	7 months	
... crawl (F) hands/knees	9 months	
... walk with one hand held	11 months	
... walk several steps	11–21 months	
... walk with 2 hands held	18 months	
... walk (B) several steps	14–15 months	
... walk 6 steps ind.	12–24 months	
... walk 10 steps unaided	24–27 months	
... walk tiptoe with demonstration—few steps	27 months	
... walk (B) 10' on a straight line	25–36 months	
... walk tiptoe 10 feet	29 months	
... walk heel/toe patterns 2 of 3 trials	44–53 months	
... walk on footprint pattern	36–48 months	
... walk (B) 4 steps—heel touching toe 2 of 3 trials	59 months	
... walk (B) (F) & (S)	48–60 months	
... tiptoe 20 or more feet	60–72 months	
BEAM/BOARD/LINE		
... one foot on walking board	20 months	
... walk on a line in a general direction	23 months	
... walk 2 steps on a		

ACTIVITIES	NORMS	COMMENTS
walking board		
...walk on a straight line 10 feet	29 months	
...walk on a walking board both feet (slide okay)	36 months	
...walk 3-inch taped line for 10 feet	42–48 months	
...walk (F) on balance beam—slide (B)	49–60 months	
...walk 1 inch taped line 10 feet	49–60 months	
...walk 1 inch pathway in 4-foot circle	49–60 months	
...walk on walking board (F) (B) (S) with no error	49–60 months	
RUN	61–72 months	
...stiffly 10 steps—eyes on ground	7–8 months	
...run (F) 10 feet—use whole foot	24–36 months	
...run around obstacles, smoothly 10 yards—coordinated	37–48 months	
...run without (F) body lean, stops, starts, change speed, turns corners quickly	49–60 months	
...runs patterns/obstacle course/50 yd	61–72 months	
...run 35 yds. in 10 seconds	61–72 months	
MISCELLANEOUS		
...march	37–48 months	
...obstacle course	49–60 months	
...slide either direction	61–72 months	
CLIMB		
...crawl up/down 2 steps	0–12 months	
...creep upstairs	15 months	
...walk up/down stairs—hold wall or rail	16 months	
...creep downstairs (B)	18–23 months	
...climb into adult chair	18 months	
...climb up/down stairs—		

ACTIVITIES	NORMS	COMMENTS
mark time without support	18–30 months	
. . . climb upstairs alternate feet	23 months	
. . . climb down stairs— alternate feet	30 months	
. . . climb large ladder mark time up/down	27–33 months	
. . . climb up ladders— alternate feet	38–47 months	
. . . climb down ladders— alternate feet	53–56 months	
. . . climb step ladder or stairs for 10 feet, effortlessly	60–72 months	

JUMP

. . . down one stair step— foot lead, land on all 4's or squat	19–24 months	
. . . in place—off the floor 2 times	22–23 months	
. . . over a line or small object	19–24 months	
. . . independently from 11" or assisted from 18"	24 months	
. . . up/over string 2" high	29+ months	
. . . down from 2nd step (14"–18")	29+ months	
. . . long jump 8½"	31 months	
. . . over string 8" high	29 months	
. . . down 28" with help	36 months	
. . . down independently 28", feet together	44 months	
. . . standing high jump 2" from crouch	48 months	
. . . standing broad jump 8–10" (2 foot usage)	48 months	
. . . over knee-high obstacle, both feet together	49–60 months	
. . . jump forward 10 times w/out falling	49–60 months	

ACTIVITIES	NORMS	COMMENTS
... jump backward 6 times w/out falling	49–60 months	
... leap over rope 10″–16″ high	49–60 months	
... standing broad jump 25″	49–60 months	
... high jump 17″	61–72 months	
... standing broad jump 38 inches	61–72 months	
... down own shoulder height	61–72 months	

HOP

... one one foot at least 2 times	29+ months	
... 10 or more steps, both feet	42 months	
... 4–6 steps, one foot	46 months	
... 2–3 yds., either foot	56–60 months	
... hop 10 times or more	55–60 months	
... hop 5 yds within 18″ alley ½ trails	61–72 months	

GALLOP-SKIP

... smoothly — 4 successive steps	48 months	

BALL SKILLS

... tracks ball or object	3 months	
... reaches for and grasps object 3–9″ in front	3 months	
... transfer object from 1 hand to other	3 months	
... puts down 1 object deliberately to reach another	3 months	
... throw or roll ball	10 months	
... rolls ball in imitation	13–24 months	
... definite fling of ball	13 months	
... throws small ball overhand 1–3′	19 months	
... kicks ball forward	13–24 months	
... rolls ball forward	25–36 months	
... throws underhand	30 months	
... throws ball to adult 5′ away, w/out		

ACTIVITIES	NORMS	COMMENTS
adult moving feet	25–36 months	
. . . catches rolled ball	25–36 months	
. . . throws ball 10′ — guide with fingers may shift weight, use shoulder and elbow with some accuracy	36–56 months	
. . . kick large ball rolled to him	37–48 months	
. . . bounces large ball 4 feet	37–48 months	
. . . catches large bounced ball with hands — 2 of 3 times, elbows extended	47–48 months	
. . . throw ball 12–18′ with good direction, poor height control	48–60 months	
. . . throw bean bag into basket	48–60 months	
. . . kicks 10″ ball toward target	48–60 months	
. . . bounce and catch large ball	48–60 months	
. . . bounce ball under control	48–60 months	
. . . chest large ball arms bending	61 months	
. . . bats balloon aloft 30 seconds	57 months	
. . . roll ball to hit object	61–72 months	
. . . throw almost adult stance	61–72 months	
. . . kick soccer ball in air 8′ 1/3 x's	61–72 months	
. . . bounces tennis ball with 1 hand and catches with 2–4/10 x's	60 months	
. . . dribbles ball with direction	60 months	
. . . catches using hands more than arms	60 months	
. . . catches soft ball or bean bag with one hand	60 months	
. . . hits (swinging) ball		

ACTIVITIES	*NORMS*	*COMMENTS*
with bat or stick	60 months	
PLAY EQUIPMENT		
. . . use rocking chair/horse	12–24 months	
. . . forward somersault		
with help	25–36 months	
. . . pedal trike 5′—steers	37–48 months	
. . . swings when started	37–48 months	
. . . climb and slides down		
5′ slide	37–48 months	
. . . roller skate 10 feet	49–60 months	
. . . pedal-turn-backwards		
on trike	49–60 months	
. . . ride bike with training		
wheels	60–72 months	
. . . slides on sled	60–72 months	
. . . steers wagon propelled		
with 1 foot	60–72 months	
. . . backward somersault	60–72 months	

GROSS MOTOR ASSESSMENT—LEVEL I

Name _____ M F Age _____ Date _____

* (−) indicates performance less than mature or incorrect

** marks time—both feet are placed on each step or in each space

when two or more phrases are separated by (/), circle appropriate one(s)

I. Locomotion and Balance   *Comments*

A. Creeps 10 feet without assistance (on hands and knees)

_____ moves forward toward object without help

_____ moves backwards without help

_____ uses contralateral (opposite hand from leg)/ ipsilateral (same side) (−)* pattern

B. Walks 20 feet without assistance

1. Forward

_____ walks with heel to toe weight transfer

_____ walks using even stride without help

_____ walks with small steps, feet wide for balance without help (−)

_____ arms swing back and forth rhythmically

_____ arms held up and/or out for balance (−)

2. Backwards

_____ walks with toe to heel weight transfer

_____ walks using even stride without help

_____ walks with small steps, feet wide for balance without help (−)

_____ arms swing back and forth rhythmically

_____ arms held up and/or out for balance (−)

C. Walks on 9″ wide walking board

1. Forward

_____ steps on without help

_____ walks without stepping off; distance travelled _____

_____ arms relaxed at sides

_____ arms held up and/or out for balance (−)

_____ steps off without help

2. Backwards

_____ steps on without help

_____ walks without stepping off; distance travelled _____

_____ arms relaxed at sides

_____ arms held up and/or out for balance (−)

_____ steps off without help

D. Walks on 9″ wide walking board placed on incline

    _____ steps on without help

    _____ walks without stepping off; distance travelled _____

    _____ arms relaxed at sides

    _____ arms held up and/or out for balance (−)

    _____ steps off without help

E. Steps into spaces of ladder lying on floor

    1. Forward

    _____ does without touching rungs

    _____ feet alternate/marks time ** (−)

    2. Backward

    _____ does without touching rungs

    _____ feet alternate/marks time ** (−)

F. Walks on 4″ wide balance beam

    1. Forward

    _____ steps on without help

    _____ walks placing one foot in front of other without stepping off; distance travelled _____

    _____ arms relaxed at sides

    _____ arms held up and/or out for balance (−)

    _____ does not have excess body motion

    _____ steps off without help

    2. Backwards

    _____ steps on without help

    _____ walks placing one foot in front of other without stepping off; distance travelled _____

    _____ arms relaxed at sides

    _____ arms held up and/or out for balance (−)

    _____ does not have excess body motion

    _____ steps off without help

G. Sits down and stands up using small chair

    _____ sits down without help

    _____ stands up without help

H. Sits down and stands up from floor

    _____ sits down without help

    _____ stands up without help

I. Bends to floor and returns to stand

    _____ bends over, picks up objects and returns to upright position without help and without falling

J. Steps down from 1-foot height

_____ steps off 1-foot-high platform without help

K. Runs

_____ runs without help; distance travelled _____

_____ runs so there is a momentary period where both feet are not in contact with floor in each stride

_____ runs with even stride/short and wide steps (−); distance travelled _____

_____ runs with heel to toe weight transfer

_____ arms swing back and forth rhythmically

_____ arms bent/straight (−)

_____ arms held up and/or out for balance

II. Climbing

A. Climbs stairs

1. Up

_____ climbs without help

_____ feet alternate/mark time (−)

_____ does without using handrail

2. Down

_____ climbs without help

_____ feet alternate/mark time (−)

_____ does without using handrail

B. Steps on rungs of ladder

_____ does while ladder is lying flat on floor without help

_____ feet alternate/mark time (−)

_____ does with ladder placed on incline without help

_____ feet alternate/mark time (−)

C. Climbs upright ladder

1. Up

_____ feet alternate/mark time (−)

2. Down

_____ feet alternate/mark time (−)

III. Ball Skills

A. Holds onto 8″ ball with 2 hands

_____ does without help; time length held _____

_____ does while sitting

_____ does while standing/walking

B. Picks up 8″ ball from floor

_____ does without help

_____ holds and walks with ball; time length held _____

C. Drops 8″ ball into box
_____ does without help

D. Holds and pushes 8″ ball away from chest
_____ does without help
_____ extends arms before releasing

E. Holds small ball in one hand while standing
_____ does without help; time length held _____

F. Picks up small ball from floor
_____ does without help
_____ holds and walks with ball; time length held
_____

G. Tosses small ball
_____ releases ball underhand/overhand/drops ball
(−)
_____ uses same hand; hand used _____
_____ does without help

H. "Kicks" stationary ball by contacting it with foot
_____ pushes ball with one foot; foot used _____
_____ walks through ball; no real awareness (−)

I. "Catches" and holds onto 8″ ball
_____ accepts ball guided/gently tossed into
body
_____ watches ball
_____ holds onto ball

IV. Play Equipment

A. Sits on push toy and pushes with feet
_____ sits on push toy without help
_____ holds on with hands without help
_____ moves forward without help
_____ moves backwards without help

B. Pushes or pulls moving toy
_____ pushes toy with handle using two hands;
distance pushed _____
_____ pulls toy with string; distance pulled _____

C. Swings
_____ sits on swing without help
_____ accepts being pushed
_____ climbs on seat without help
_____ climbs off seat without help

D. Slides
_____ climbs up without help
_____ slides down without help; size of
slide _____

E. Uses seesaw

_____ accepts sitting on moving seesaw without help
_____ climbs on seat without help
_____ climbs off seat without help

F. Uses tricycle
_____ sits on stationary cycle without help
_____ accepts sitting on moving cycle without help
_____ climbs on without help
_____ climbs off without help
_____ keeps feet on pedals of moving cycle without help
_____ holds onto handlebars without help
_____ pushes pedals without help

V. Disequilibrium Equipment

A. Sits on rocking board
_____ accepts being rocked without climbing off
_____ holds on and/or leans body to stop from sliding off

B. Lies on stomach on rocking board
_____ accepts being rocked without climbing off
_____ holds on and/or leans body to stop from sliding off

C. Accepts being on trampoline
_____ creeps on trampoline mat without help
_____ walks on trampoline mat without help
_____ accepts being bounced in prone/supine position(s)
_____ accepts being bounced in sitting/creeping position(s)
_____ accepts being bounced in standing position
_____ bounces in standing position with/without holding on

VI. Interaction skills

_____ accepts and responds to interactions initiated by adult
_____ initiates interactions with adult
_____ accepts peer playing alongside/shows interest in peer
_____ accepts/responds to interaction initiated by peer

GROSS MOTOR ASSESSMENT—LEVEL II

Name _____ M F Age _____ Date _____

* (−) indicates performance less than mature or incorrect
** marks time — both feet are placed on each step or in each space
# when two or more phrases are separated by (/), circle appropriate one(s)

I. Balance   *Comments*

A. Walks on 9" wide walking board
   1. Forward
   _____ walks entire length without stepping off
   _____ uses arms to maintain balance (−)
   _____ arms remain relaxed at sides
   _____ has excess body motion (−)
   2. Backwards
   _____ walks entire length without stepping off
   _____ uses arms to maintain balance (−)
   _____ arms remain relaxed at sides
   _____ has excess body motion (−)
   3. Raised
   _____ walks with/without help
   _____ uses arms to maintain balance (−)
   _____ arms remain relaxed at sides
   _____ has excess body motion (−)

B. Walks on 4" wide balance beam
   1. Forward
   _____ steps on without help
   _____ walks entire length without stepping off; dis-
         tance travelled _____
   _____ walks placing one foot in front of other
   _____ walks using small/large steps
   _____ arms relaxed/up and out for balance (−)
   _____ has excess body motion (−)
   _____ steps off at end without help
   2. Backwards
   _____ steps on without help
   _____ walks entire length without stepping off; dis-
         tance travelled _____
   _____ walks placing one foot behind other
   _____ walks using small/large steps
   _____ arms relaxed/up and out for balance (−)
   _____ has excess body motion (−)
   _____ steps off at end without help

C. Steps into spaces of ladder lying on floor
   1. Forward
   _____ does without touching rungs
   _____ feet alternate/mark time (–)
   2. Backwards
   _____ does without touching rungs
   _____ feet alternate/mark time (–)

D. Stands on one foot
   1. Preferred foot _____
   length of time _____
   _____ has excess motion and/or clamps non-support
      leg against support leg (–)
   2. Non-preferred foot _____
   length of time _____
   _____ has excess motion and/or clamps non-support
      leg against support leg (–)

E. Crosses midline of body using crossover step
   _____ starts with feet on same side of rope
   _____ steps across rope alternating feet
   _____ steps next to rope, toes pointing straight
      ahead
   _____ maintains balance

II. Climbing

A. Climbs stairs
   1. Up
   _____ feet alternate/mark time (–)
   _____ does without using handrail
   2. Down
   _____ feet alternate/mark time (–)
   _____ does without using handrail

B. Climbs ladder
   1. Up
   _____ feet alternate/mark time (–)
   2. Down
   _____ feet alternate/mark time (–)

III. Play Equipment

A. Climbs on jungle gym
   _____ does without help; height climbed _____

B. Plays on swing
   _____ pushes with feet (–)
   _____ pumps legs

C. Plays on seesaw

_____ stays seated when his end is raised

_____ accepts up and down movement

_____ pushes with feet to raise his end

D. Plays on slide

_____ climbs up without help

_____ slides down without help

E. Rides tricycle

_____ keeps feet on pedals

_____ pushes pedals

_____ steers

F. Rides bike

_____ does with training wheel

_____ maintains balance without training wheels

_____ steers

_____ uses brakes

IV. Locomotor and Body Projection

A. Runs

_____ runs so there is a momentary period where both feet are not in contact with floor in each stride

_____ runs with even stride

_____ runs with heel to toe weight transfer

_____ arms are bent/straight (−)

_____ arms swing back and forth rhythmically

B. Slides

1. preferred lead _____

_____ moves sideways with uneven rhythm

_____ has step-close-step action

_____ has momentary period where both feet are off of floor in each-step-close step cycle

2. non-preferred lead _____

_____ moves sideways with uneven rhythm

_____ has step-close-step action

_____ has momentary period where both feet are off of floor in each step-close-step cycle

C. Gallops

1. preferred lead _____

_____ faces direction travelling with uneven rhythm

_____ has step-close-step action

_____ has momentary period where both feet are off of floor in each step-close-step cycle

2. non-preferred lead _____
_____ faces direction travelling with uneven rhythm
_____ has step-close-step action
_____ has momentary period where both feet are
off of floor in each step-close-step cycle

D. Skips
_____ gallops (−)
_____ lame duck skip (−)
_____ has step-hop pattern
_____ has smooth, uneven rhythm
_____ feet recover close to floor
_____ arms relaxed and swing freely at sides in
opposition to legs

E. Jumps off 2-foot-high raised platform
_____ takes off from two feet/one foot (−)
_____ lands on two feet/one foot (−)
_____ falls when landing (−)
_____ swings arms forward and/or up at takeoff
_____ uses arms for balance only (−)

F. Jumps over stationary rope
_____ takes off from two feet/one foot (−)
_____ lands on two feet/one foot (-)
_____ falls when landing (−)
_____ swings arms forward and/or up at takeoff
_____ uses arms for balance only (−)
_____ jumps just high enough to clear obstacle

G. Jumps over moving rope
_____ takes off from two feet/one foot (−)
_____ lands on two feet/one foot (−)
_____ falls when landing (−)
_____ swings arms forward and/or up at takeoff
_____ uses arms for balance only (−)
_____ jumps just high enough to clear obstacle

H. Jumps over series of stationary obstacles
_____ takes off from two feet/one foot (−)
_____ lands on two feet/one foot (−)
_____ falls when landing (−)
_____ swings arms forward and/or up at takeoff
_____ uses arms for balance only (−)
_____ jumps just high enough to clear obstacle
_____ has continuous rhythm

I. Performs standing long jump
_____ takes off from two feet/one foot (−)
_____ lands on two feet/one foot (−)
_____ falls when landing (−)

_____ swings arms forward at takeoff

_____ extends arms/body forward at takeoff distance jumped _____

J. Performs hopscotch

_____ has two feet-one foot-two feet pattern

_____ remains within boxes

K. Hops

1. Preferred foot _____

   non-support leg position: _____ in front of support leg

   _____ behind support leg

   _____ uses non-support leg in pumping action

   _____ arms swing in opposition/swing up and/or out (−)

   number of consecutive hops _____

2. Non-preferred foot _____

   non-support leg position: _____ in front of support leg

   _____ behind support leg

   _____ uses non-support leg in pumping action

   _____ arms swing in opposition/swing up and/or out (−)

   number of consecutive hops _____

V. Ball Skills

A. Throws using 2-hand chest pass

_____ holds ball at chest using 2 hands

_____ pushes ball away from chest by extending arms

_____ steps forward and shifts weight forward

_____ throws to partner so can be caught _____ feet away

B. Throws overhand with _____ hand

_____ cocks hand overhead

_____ releases ball overhand

_____ steps forward onto _____ foot and shifts weight forward

_____ has body rotation

_____ has preparatory wind up of throwing arm

_____ throws to partner so can be caught _____ feet away

C. Throws underhand with _____ hand

_____ has backswing of throwing arm

_____ releases ball underhand

_____ steps forward onto _____ foot and transfers weight forward

_____ throws to partner so can be caught _____ feet away

D. Rolls ball with _____ hand

_____ has backswing of throwing arm

_____ releases ball so it rolls on floor

_____ steps forward onto _____ foot and bends knees

_____ rolls so hits target _____ feet away

E. Catches ball

_____ watches ball

_____ reaches ball with both hands as it comes to body

_____ catches with hands/traps ball (–)

_____ catches large/medium/small balls

F. Catches ball not tossed directly to him

_____ watches ball

_____ reaches ball with both hands as it comes to body

_____ catches with hands/traps ball (–)

_____ catches large/medium/small balls

_____ moves body in line with tossed ball

G. Kicks stationary ball with _____ foot

_____ takes running/walking approach, 3 steps minimum

_____ does not pause to kick ball

_____ makes solid contact with ball; kicks hard

H. Kicks rolling ball with _____ foot

_____ takes running/walking approach, 3 steps minimum

_____ does not pause to kick ball

_____ makes solid contact with ball; kicks hard

I. Drops and catches large ball using two hands

_____ drops and catches ball after one bounce

J. Dribbles ball

1. preferred hand _____

_____ dribbles in place

_____ dribbles while walking/running

_____ keeps ball under control, no higher than chest level

_____ hand pushes ball down to floor

   2. non-preferred hand _____
_____ dribbles in place
_____ dribbles while walking/running
_____ keeps ball under control, no higher than
      chest level
_____ hand pushes ball down to floor

K. Using whiffle bat, bats _____ handed
_____ has parallel stance
_____ swings bat so arms extended at contact
_____ follows through with bat
_____ transfers weight onto forward foot
_____ makes solid contact with ball
_____ hits medium/small ball off batting tee
_____ hits medium/small ball tossed underhand

L. Uses plastic hockey stick and puck
_____ can hit puck to partner
_____ stops puck hit to him
_____ dribbles puck

M. Shoots basketball
_____ uses 2-hand/1-hand shoot
_____ makes lay-ups
_____ makes set shots

VI. Trampoline

_____ bounces on feet remaining on cross +
_____ performs check bounce (bounce and stop)
_____ bounces on knees
_____ performs knee drop
_____ performs seat drop
_____ performs 4-point (hands and knees) drop
_____ performs front drop
_____ performs 1/4, 1/2, 3/4, full turns
_____ performs tuck/pike/straddle bounce
      performs stunt combinations:

VII. Interaction skills

_____ accepts/responds to adult-initiated inter-
      actions
_____ initiates interactions with adult
_____ accepts/responds to peer-initiated interaction
_____ initiates interactions with peers
_____ plays parallel/cooperatively/competitively

GROSS MOTOR ASSESSMENT—LEVEL III
(assess skills in Level II, then assess game concepts)

I. Game Concepts   *Comments*

A. Kickball/baseball

_____ knows names of bases

_____ runs bases in correct order, touching each base

_____ hits ball and runs to first base

_____ understands concepts of "safe" and "out"

_____ runs to next base when another player hits ball

_____ knows when to advance more than one base without being put out

_____ understands concept of foul ball

_____ understands concepts regarding caught fly ball: hitter is out/base runners must tag up at original base

_____ knows how to field ball and throw to baseman to get runner out

_____ knows how to play first base

B. Soccer/floor hockey/basketball

_____ understands how to shoot for goal and score points

_____ passes ball/puck to teammate appropriately

_____ will retrieve loose ball/puck

_____ receives pass and shoots for goal

_____ understands concept of player-to-player defense against opponent

_____ understands difference between defending own goal and attacking opponent's goal

GROSS MOTOR ASSESSMENT REPORT—LEVEL I

Name: Jesse
Age: 5 years
Reporter: Kim

Jesse was assessed at the ISDD using a non-standardized gross motor checklist. He was cooperative during the assessment and did not fuss at all. Jesse needed to be guided to most activities in order to ensure that he got them, as he was distracted easily.

In the area of balance, Jesse had highs and lows. The most obvious high was his ability to balance himself on the edge of mats or other high "seats" and not fall. He also walked up and down a 9″ wide board on an incline and on the floor, independently. He shuffled very slowly. He stepped in the spaces of a ladder on the floor in a mark time manner. On the 4″ wide beam, Jesse wanted to hold on to me or something; if he did not have anything to hold, he stopped and would not move. Yet when he held onto me, he did not cling and seemed very much at ease. When I had Jesse stand on a vestibular (rocking) board, he was somewhat frightened when I let go. His eyes widened, arms went out and he bent at the waist. He immediately got down on all fours and off of the board. Jesse did run, but not consistently upon direction. He had his eyes to the ground and ran 10′–15′ before he stopped. He was inconsistently flat-footed or on his toes. Jesse climbed up and down stairs independently when holding onto a handrail. He used an alternate foot pattern going up and a mark time pattern going down. He climbed on the inclined ladder with a mark time pattern going up and needed total assistance to get down.

Jesse did not jump, even on a mini-tramp. He used a stepdown movement from any height and had to be assisted to do that.

Upper/lower extremity control was checked using ball skills. Jesse would track a ball by turning his head, not just his eyes; he would reach and grasp small balls, transfer hand to hand, throw small balls 1′–3′ forward using his right hand, or use both hands to toss a playground ball out 3′ independently. Jesse kicked independently only after he was physically assisted to kick the first ball and then moved into place to kick the rest. He put bean bags into a basket that was moved from side to side or up and down. Jesse did not catch balls tossed or rolled to him, but he did reach out and appear to watch for them. If a ball went to either side, he made no attempt to get it.

Jesse can get on a trike and put his feet on the pedals when given cues, but not pedal.

Recommendations

In order to learn skills, Jesse needs an adapted physical education program that follows a consistent structured routine. He will learn best by repetition of the desired skills over a period of time.

Balance skills such as walking on balance beams, walking board that are flat on the floor or on an incline would help Jesse.

Have him run to an object or a person. Use his favorite toy as a reinforcer.

Practice jumping on a mini-tramp and then in place. Work on stepping down from 12″ independently.

Throw and roll balls to a target. Use his hands to catch a rolled ball or gently tossed ball. Kick stationary balls and shoot baskets into boxes or wastebaskets.

Sit on and pedal a trike with physical assistance.

Implementors: Adapted Physical Education
Annual Goal: Jesse will perform a variety of movement activities

Short-term objectives	Amount of Time	Methods and Materials	Evaluation Procedures	Criteria	Date Achieved
a. Jesse will walk the entire length of the 9" board on the floor independently	P.E.	Verbal cues, demonstration, physical assistance	Daily logs	5 of 5 times	
b. Jesse will throw a medium (8") or small (3") ball to an adult or target 3–4 feet away.	P.E.	Verbal cues, demonstration, physical assistance	Daily logs	4 of 5 times	
c. Jesse will walk the entire length of the 4" balance beam independently.	P.E.	Verbal cues, demonstration, physical assistance	Daily logs	3 of 5 times	
d. Jesse will run 10' without assistance with one verbal cue to stand in a more upright position.	P.E.	Verbal cues, demonstration, physical assistance	Daily logs	4 of 5 times	
e. Jesse will jump using a 2-foot takeoff and landing in a designated area.	P.E.	Verbal cues, demonstration, physical assistance	Daily logs	3 of 5 times	

Student: _____ Lesson # _____ Date: _____ Time: _____

Objective/Activity	Important Points and Procedures	Evaluation of Lesson
Climbing	Climb up and down stairs marking time independently Climb up and down ladder placed on incline, keeping feet on rungs	
Balance moving forward	Walk across 9″ walking board independently, when raised Walk across 4″ balance beam independently	
Balance moving backward	Walk across 9″ walking board independently Step into the space of a ladder on the floor	
Jumping from platform	Jump down from various heights (6″–2′) using 2-foot takeoff and landing	
Jumping from spot to spot spot to another	Using 2-foot takeoff: landing to move from one marked	
Locomotor slide	Use step/close/step pattern with minimal assistance	
Ball skills		
Chest pass	Throw a medium-size ball using 2 hands starting ball at chest level into a large box	
Overhand	Throw a small ball using dominant hand to target on wall, remaining inside a hoop on the floor	
Kick	A stationary ball using 3-step approach	
Catch	A medium-size ball that is gently tossed to him from a distance of 3–5 feet.	
Play equipment		
Tricycle	Sit on and pedal a trike for	

Objective/Activity	Important Points and Procedures	Evaluation of Lesson
	a minimum of one minute	
Swing	Sit on and attempt to push swing with feet	
Scooter	Sit on and move forward, backward, etc., for at least 30 seconds	

GOAL: **Jesse will perform a variety of movement activities.**

Objective A: Jesse will walk the entire length of the 9" wide board on the floor, independently.

Procedure: Say: "Jesse, walk on the board," and while holding his hand, direct him to the end of the board. Restate the direction. If he hesitates, physically assist on to the board.

Objective B: Jesse will throw a medium (8") or small (3") ball to an adult or target 3–4 feet away.

Procedure: Say: "Jesse, throw the ball to me." Squat five feet from Jesse with outstretched arms indicating where he should throw the ball. If he hesitates, repeat the direction and physically assist him to throw the ball. A target could be a box, hoop, wastepaper basket or clothes basket.

Objective C: Jesse will walk the entire length of the 4" balance beam.

Procedure: Same as A above.

Objective D: Jesse will run ten feet without assistance in a more upright position, with one verbal cue.

Procedure: Say: "Jesse, run over to the window." Point to the window and give the direction. If he hesitates, take Jesse's hand and assist him partway. If still hesitant, run with Jesse the entire length.

Objective E: Jesse will jump using a 2-foot takeoff and landing in a designated area.

Procedure: Say: "Jesse, jump off the (mats)." Demonstrate first and if he hesitates, restate the direction and physically assist through the movement.

Objective F: Jesse will ride a tricycle independently for 30 feet.

Procedure: Say: "Jesse, it's time to ride the bike." Help him to get on and sit. Push down on his raised knee to help initiate the pedalling motion.

GROSS MOTOR ASSESSMENT REPORT—LEVEL II

Name: Matt
Age: 10 years
Reporter: Kim Davis

Matt's gross motor skills were assessed during an observation time that included a variety of activities designed to allow Matt to play and move as independently as possible.

On the 9″ wide walking board, Matt easily walked forward and backward the entire length. He was not sure of a raised board (2′), but did cross a board 7 inches off the floor very easily. On a 4″ wide beam, he got halfway across before he stepped off. His arms were relaxed and he placed one foot ahead of the other to move. He refused to walk backward on the 4″ beam.

When directed to step into the spaces of a ladder on the floor, he consistently stepped on the rungs but used alternating feet.

He did not successfully stand on one foot; he could not stand still and, therefore, one foot balance is difficult. He stood on the edge of a hula hoop placed on the ground to help him orient himself and his "space," rather than inside it.

Matt marked time when climbing up the inclined ladder in the room.

Matt does run with feet off the floor and some heel to toe weight transfer. His stride is somewhat uneven, but he does use his arms bent at the elbow and swinging at his sides.

Jumping down/over/out were all problems due more to behavior of refusal than ability. He stepped off a 7″ high platform and over a stationary rope or series of ropes. He stepped over and then added a little hopping motion after he was across the ropes. He did use a 2-foot takeoff/landing when told to jump out as far as he could. He jumped 2 feet. He could jump vertically, approximately 6″ off the floor. He did not use his arms, but did bend his knees.

Hopping was difficult for him. He did attempt but could not do the movement.

Matt did throw small balls with his left hand by bending his elbow and pitching the balls 5′–8′. He used no weight shift, body rotation, or stride feet. He rolled a bowling ball with his left hand at pins 4′ away. He did not use any preparatory movement prior to the roll.

When catching balls, Matt will more often hit the balls away rather than catch them. He did watch and reach out for the balls. When he did catch, he trapped the balls against his body.

He used his left foot to kick but was inconsistent, especially with balls rolled to him. When rolled, he used whatever foot the ball was closer to at that time. He did not make solid contact.

Matt had difficulty with body control when bouncing and catching a ball or dribbling.

He held a wiffle bat (right-handed) given a demonstration. With it he hit a medium-size ball off a batting tee. He did follow all the way around with the bat, but his body control, weight shift, rotation, etc., were poor.

Matt will march and do motions to music for short periods of time with the group.

Matt seemed very unsure of how to do many activities due to lack of exposure to them. His behavior is possibly also a big part of his apparent inability to locate body parts or move in directed ways.

Recommendations

Matt needs a directed gross motor program that includes a variety of skills for him to learn.

The use of ball skills in purposeful play activities would be beneficial. Simple games that involved a few other players would enhance his motor and social skills.

Body awareness, body parts and spatial relations could be learned in simple games such as Follow the Leader, Simon Says or through the use of music and aerobic exercise.

Implementors: Adapted Physical Education
Annual Goal: Matt will improve and use gross motor skills in purposeful activity

Short-term objectives	Amount of Time	Methods and Materials	Evaluation Procedures	Criteria	Date Achieved
a. Matt will develop ball skills, throw, kick, roll, catch, for simple games	P.E.	Verbal cues, demonstration, physical assistance	Daily logs	3 of 10 times each skill	
b. Matt will use running in a constructive game (tag, race).	P.E.	Verbal cues, demonstration, physical assistance	Daily logs	3 of 10 times when situation arises	
c. Matt will learn body parts and different ways to move (dance exercise).	P.E.	Verbal cues, demonstration, physical assistance	Daily logs	3 of 10 times when asked	
d. Matt will swim a distance of 20 feet from one person to another.	P.E.	Verbal cues, demonstration, physical assistance	Daily logs	3 of 5 times when asked	

Student: _____ Lesson # _____ Date: _____ Time: _____

Objective/Activity	Important Points and Procedures	Evaluation of Lesson

Simple Ball Games
  Floor Hockey   Initially passing
  Soccer   ball or puck to partner, then
                       to target, and finally receive
                       a pass and shoot for a goal
  Basketball   Add dribbling in basketball
  Bowling   Bowl with adult for 3
                       complete turns each, with
                       two rolls per turn
  "Tee" Ball   Initially hit 6 balls of tee
                       and circle bases between
                       hits
                       Next adult fields the ball
                       and tells her to get around
                       the bases before adult can
                       tag him
  Kickball   Once the concept is
                       understood, introduce
                       kickball

All is to be done *gradually,* not all at once

Exercises
  Situps   Demonstrate a day ahead of
  Toe Touch   time and tell her it will not
  Arm Circle   be a choice tomorrow
  Trunk Twist   Initially 5 repetitiions of
                       1 exercise a day
                       When she is doing all
                       comfortable, have her do 2
                       of the 5 repetitions each

Gradual increases and changes explained ahead of time are vital

GOAL: Matt will improve and use gross motor skills in purposeful activity.

Objective A: Matt will develop ball skills such as throwing, kicking, rolling, and catching for simple game activities.

Procedure: Work on each skill individually at first, then combine them. For throwing and rolling set up targets to throw to (posters, bowling pins, boxes). Place a hoop, carpet square or "X" on the floor for him to throw from. (This will help with spatial problems and keep him from walking up and placing the balls in/on the targets.)

Demonstrate and tell him exactly what to do. Give him time. He needs time and space to feel comfortable.

For kicking, place balls (large-medium size) on bean bags to help hold them still. Demonstrate and tell him exactly what he is to do. For catching, initially use nerf or beach ball and toss them gently. Gradually increase the distance and use of other smaller/harder balls.

Objective B: Matt will use running in a constructive game (tag, races, etc.)

Procedure: Place activities Matt likes at one end of the room and tell him he may play with them if he races or runs with the adult present. Do not let him have the activities unless he runs. Gradually increase the distance or times he runs across the room before reinforcement. Playing chase or tag can be rewarding in itself. He likes to be caught and swung around.

Objective C: Matt will learn body parts and different ways to move, dance, exercise, march, relax, etc.

Procedure: Name and point to body parts and have Matt repeat them. If he does not talk, accept a pointing or touching of the correct body part. As he progresses, use cards with body parts to name, or put together a flannel board with body parts.

With the use of music, demonstrate and encourage Matt to march, dance or "move" to the music.

As he grows more comfortable and trusting, have him lie down on mats to do simple exercises such as sit-ups, toe touches, and leg lifts. Also practice some relaxation by tightening and loosening the muscles in his arms and legs.

Objective D: Matt will swim a distance of 20 feet from one person to another.

Procedure: Matt will be allowed to become comfortable and play in the water before the adult requests him to do anything. The adult will approach Matt in a playful manner and try to get him to imitate movements such as diving underwater or jumping up and down. He will then be given a kickboard and asked to swim with it, with time alone being the reinforcer. Any distance he swims will be accepted at first.

GROSS MOTOR ASSESSMENT REPORT—LEVEL III

Name: Sara
Age: 11
Reporter: Kim

Sara's gross motor skills were assessed using an observational checklist that includes a variety of motor skills. The assessment room was arranged to allow Sara the maximum use of all of the equipment.

Sara had no difficulty crossing the 4″ and 9″ wide balance beams while walking forward. She refused to walk backward on the beams, but did walk backward on a footprint pattern on the floor independently. She did need a demonstration to understand the directions. She did stand on one foot to balance and her right foot seemed to be her preferred side.

She had no problem climbing stairs, ladders, or jungle gyms.

Sara had an age-appropriate running pattern. When given a model and a footprint pattern on the floor to follow, she was able to slide. However, she faced forward and used gliding motion, as in skating. When she was given a model for gallop, she skipped. Her skip was a "lame duck" skip which alternates with a true skip step/hop motion. She was stiff and used her arms very little.

Sara's jumping skills were not consistent in her use of a two-foot takeoff and landing. There were times she leaped instead of jumped, landing on one foot rather than two. She did jump down/out and over objects and maintained her balance. She had limited arm use for assistance in movement. To jump over a series of objects, she used a leaping motion. Sara did hop on her right foot as her preferred foot. She held her non-supporting leg behind and had limited arm movement.

Sara used her right side as her dominant side. She tossed small balls to an adult or target 6′ away with only arm use. She had little rotation or weight shift. Rolling a bowling ball was done right-handed with a backswing, but inconsistent release on the floor. She watched and reached for balls tossed to her and inconsistently trapped medium/small balls against her body. She could drop and catch a ball and dribble a ball while stationary or moving with some amount of control. She kicked stationary or moving balls with her right foot with inconsistent contact. She used 2 hands to shoot for baskets, used her right hand to hold a wiffle bat and hit balls off a batting tee. She was awkward with the bat.

Recommendations

Sara needs a structured gross motor time to practice the many skills that she has presently. By refining her skills, she would be better able to play on the playground or in physical education classes with her peers.

Use actual sports or games to practice ball skills so she learns that they have a meaning and how they are used in each game.

Develop playground skills such as jump rope, hopscotch or tag games.

Begin a simple exercise and movement program to help maintain some level of fitness.

Make the class reinforcing to Sara so she enjoys what she is doing and wants to work while in physical education.

Implementors: Adapted Physical Education
Annual Goal: Sara will use her gross motor skills and apply them in sports and game situations.

Short-term objectives	Amount of Time	Methods and Materials	Evaluation Procedures	Criteria	Date Achieved
a. Sara will use ball skills (throw, catch, kick, roll) in simple games or sports activities such as croquet, floor hockey, etc.	P.E.	Verbal cues, demonstration, physical assistance	Daily logs	8 out of 10 times a game or sport is played, she will be successful	
b. Sara will use skills of jumping, hopping, skipping, running in games, races, jump rope and other playground type games	P.E.	Verbal cues, demonstration, physical assistance	Daily logs	6 out of 10 times activity presented she will be successful	
c. Sara will learn and do simple exercises given only verbal cues.	P.E.	Verbal cues	Daily logs	10 out of 10 times the exercise is presented, she will comply	
d. Sara will learn and imitate simple movements to music	P.E.	Verbal cues, demonstration, physical assistance	Daily logs	6 out of 10 times presented, she will comply	
e. Sara will work on activities in the AAHPER-Kennedy Foundation Special Fitness test to earn awards (7 activities)	P.E.	Verbal cues, demonstration, physical assistance		Will reach criterion on each activity	
f. Sara will roller skate independently using a gliding motion	P.E.	Verbal cues, demonstration, physical assistance	Daily logs	8 feet 3 times	

g. Sara will ride a small two-wheeled bike for 6 feet with initial support only	P.E.	Verbal cues, demon-stration, physical assistance	Daily logs	4 of 5 times
h. Sara will front float with a kick board and blow bubbles while supported by an adult.	P.E.	Verbal cues, demon-stration, physical assistance	Daily logs	3 feet, 3 out of 5 times

Student: _____ Lesson # _____ Date: _____ Time: _____

Objective/Activity	Important Points and Procedures	Evaluation of Lesson
Ball Skills—	Use sports such as croquet, bowling, floor hockey,	
Throw—Catch Roll—Kick Bat—Dribble	soccer, kickball, baseball, basketball, volleyball, 4-square to practice the skills. Stay with one sport skill for an extended amount of time. Throw to target, kick to target, roll to target, catch using hands/feet, use bat/hockey stick to hit ball/puck to partner	
Playground Skills Jump—hop—run	Hopscotch—initially only pattern on the floor, later include the tossing "rock" skills Higher and lower—tag—"It" wears hat or carries something to distinguish self—races	
Exercises	Sit-ups—toe touches—arm circles—shuttle run	
Rhythm	Singing/movement games—use record for clapping/stomping to music	
Fitness Test	7 Activities: sit-ups—arm hang—shuttle run—standing broad jump—(SBJ)—50-yard dash—softball throw—300-yard walk/run	

GOAL: Sara will use her gross motor skills and apply them in sports and game situations.

Objective A: Sara will use ball skills (throw, catch, kick, roll) in simple games or sports activities such as croquet, floor hockey, etc.

Procedure: The remainder of games on the list are basketball, baseball, kickball, soccer, volleyball, bowling, and four-square. The skill of throwing, which is used in basketball, baseball, and kickball, should be practiced with the appropriate balls when possible. For small balls, a one-hand throw is to be used, with larger balls two-hand overhead or chest passes are to be used. Practice throwing to adult or target 8–15 feet away accurately. If she needs instruction on proper foot placement the use of footprints in stride position can help guide her. Talk about the different games that use throwing skills. Catching should also be practiced with the appropriate ball. Emphasize looking and reaching for the ball. Toss the balls gently from close distances initially. As she improves with different sizes, increase the distances of the tosses and also add bounces to some of the tosses. That would be practice on catching bounce passes as in basketball.

Kicking is used in soccer and kickball. Practice with appropriate balls. Set up a target or goal 10–15 feet away and have her kick stationary balls to the goal. When she is consistently hitting the target, roll the ball to her and have her kick to the target. Next, play "catch," kicking the ball back and forth. Another step would be to have her kick as far as she can and run around bases while the adult or another child chases the ball. Finally, have her control her kicking as in dribbling a soccer ball across the room.

Rolling is involved in bowling. Set up the pins or a target 10′–15′ away. If a rubber/plastic bowling ball is used, have Sara place her fingers in the proper holes. Use tape of footprints to have her feet in a stride position facing the pins. Let her attempt one roll; if she has difficulty, demonstrate for her and talk her through the movement. If she will allow it, physically assist her through the movement. Stand beside her and gently swing her arm. Count 1–2–3, backswing, forward, release. Have her count and write down the number of pins knocked down.

Other skills which may be tried are bouncing and dribbling balls as in four-square and basketball. This should be done with appropriate ball, two-handed initially, going to one hand as she chooses. Volleying or hitting ball in the air (volleyball) should be practiced initially with beach balls or balloons due to their slow movement. Demonstrate and practice hitting to self or to partner. Hitting balls with sports equipment, such as bats, croquet mallets, or floor hockey sticks, should be done with stationary balls/pucks initially. Gradually adding movement to the balls and pucks will inhibit frustration. The use of a batting tee to practice for baseball/softball is excellent. Stress hitting to a specific location or goal for hockey and croquet. Demonstrate all skills for her at first.

Objective B: Sara will use skills of jumping, hopping, skipping and running in games, races, jump rope and other playground games.

Procedure: Some games to be tried: hopscotch, higher and lower, racing and tag. Prior to each game an explanation will be needed to tell her exactly what will be happening and what she will be trying to do.

Hopscotch involves hopping and jumping skills. There are a number of patterns for hopscotch. Our pattern will be tried initially; later on modified patterns may be tried. In the beginning merely work on the jump/hop movements. Once she has mastered those and can move in a controlled fashion, introduce the throwing of the rock onto the numbers in the sequence and not touching that square with her foot.

Higher and Lower is a jump rope game with the rope held on the floor and gradually raised. If no other people are available to hold the ends, the rope can be tied to a chair, pole, table leg, etc., at one or both ends. Gradually move the rope higher. Jumps or running leaps over the rope are acceptable.

Racing will have to be explained clearly, and definitive starting and finishing points will need to be marked. Possibly place some motivating object at the finish line that can be obtained by the winner. Allow for Sara's success in the beginning. Gradually add more speed and/or distance to the races or make up relays. Tag will probably be the most difficult game for Sara. "It" needs to be someone/thing concrete and visible at first. Someone to avoid, yet not to run totally away from. Playing tag inside within set boundaries would be the best place to start the skill. Possibly having "It" wear a hat or hold something in the early stages would help with identification.

Objective C: Sara will learn and do simple exercises given only verbal cues.

Procedure: The exercises to be done are: sit-ups, toe touches, trunk twister, leg lifts, arm circles, and arm lifts with light weights. All exercises should be demonstrated for Sara before she is to do them.

Objective D: Sara will learn and imitate simple movements to music.

Procedure: Using singing games, demonstrate movement for Sara to imitate, clapping, swaying, stamping feet etc. Possibly work in some simple dance steps from aerobic dance at a slower pace. There are records with music and vocalization to explore different movement patterns which would be helpful for Sara.

Objective E: Sara will work on activities in the AAHPER—Kennedy Foundation Special Fitness Test to earn awards.

Procedure: The seven activities involved are sit-ups, flexed arm hang, shuttle run, standing broad jump, 50-yard dash, softball throw and 300-yard walk/run. Demonstrate all activities for Sara and participate with her to help keep her encouraged. To earn awards, children have to do a certain number of the exercises and finish within a set time. A chart will be kept of her progress.

Objective F: Sara will roller skate independently using a gliding motion.

Procedure: Sara should make an attempt to put her skates on herself: put foot into skate, tighten with key and fasten strap. Demonstrate first if needed. Assist only after she has tried first herself.

Start on carpeted surface; next go to smooth surface with Sara holding onto adult. Have Sara skate 2 or 3 feet to adult on smooth surface. She may be anxious about falling. Acknowledge her fears and reassure her. Gradually increase distance and fade adult assistance.

To teach the gliding motion, have Sara hold onto waist of adult while adult demonstrates gliding motion in an exaggerated way. Have Sara imitate. Next have her imitate gliding motion while holding one hand of an adult. Fade adult.

Objective G: Sara will ride a small 2-wheel bike for six feet with initial support only.

Procedure: Begin with a 22″ bike. Adult holds onto back of seat. Guide handlebars only as needed. Gradually reduce support as Sara improves her balance.

Objective H: Sara will front float with a kick and blowing bubbles.

Procedure: Demonstrate holding onto side and kicking. Have Sara imitate. Demonstrate blowing bubbles and have her imitate. Put both steps together and have her imitate.

As Sara holds onto side with kick, gradually add adult support. Place hand under Sara's stomach (ask permission first), have her hold onto adult with one hand and the side with the other hand. Gradually have her let go of side and hold onto adult so she can move through water in prone position with kick.

BEHAVIOR PLAN

Behavior	Antecedent	Intervention/Consequence
Mildly aggressive (pinching)	Upset Frustrated	A. If he pinches —If he pinches: sit out. (Allow processing time—use gestures.) "I'll count to 3 then help you." Count aloud and show fingers. 1,2,3 (help if needed). Set time for 2 minutes. If calm, return to activity; if not, set timer for 2 additional minutes. B. If he needs physical assistance to stay in/sit out —Give one warning, "Stay in/sit out or you go to Time Out." —If he continues to aggress and/or doesn't stay in/sit out, put in Time Out for 5 minutes. —If calm, return to activity. If not, set timer for additional 5 minutes.
Biting hand and pressing on adult's face	Happy	Say, "Do you want to shake hands?" and hold out your hand as if to shake. Give him a choice; don't force him to shake your hand.
Biting hand and pressing on adult's face	Frustrated	Say, "Tell me." If he says, "move" and you can't move, say "First _____; then I'll move."
Refusal to eat something	Doesn't like	Ignore if getting a variety of foods. Monitor food intake. Use a contingency, "First eat a bite of _____, then cracker, etc."
Not eating at dinner	When he is overactive	Expect him to sit at table for 10 minutes before he is excused.
Moving food off his plate	Doesn't like	Told to keep food on his plate.
Use of	Likes	Remind him how much he gets before

Behavior	Antecedent	Intervention/Consequence
Condiments		he pours.
Inappropriate talking	Self-stimulation Attention	Redirect to something appropriate in a positive way, such as: repeating sequence of task, reminder of "We're talking about _____."
Refusal to move and/or shoving	"His mind is set" on a routine. Unsure of what is expected.	Let him know expectation. Give him warnings, i.e., "In 3 minutes we are going to _____." In 1 minute,_____," etc. Give him as much routine as possible. Expect him to participate. Use count (1,2,3, . . .) and make sure he completes the task.

Appendix C

SPORTS SKILLS CHECKLISTS

Bowling Skills

_____ CARRIES OWN BALL TO THE LINE
_____ PUSHES BALL _____ SITTING _____ STANDING
_____ USES 2 HANDS TO ROLL/PUSH
_____ USES 1 HAND TO ROLL/PUSH
_____ KEEPS FINGERS IN PROPER ALIGNMENT/HOLES
_____ SWINGS ARM BACK THEN FORWARD (FOLLOW THROUGH)
_____ PLACES OPPOSITE FOOT AT LINE
_____ STATIONARY DELIVERY
_____ WALKS INTO DELIVERY _____ RUNNING DELIVERY
_____ STAYS BEHIND FOUL LINE
_____ REPORTS NUMBER OF PINS DOWN
_____ KNOWS EACH PERSON HAS 2 ROLLS
_____ UNDERSTANDS GUTTER BALL
_____ UNDERSTANDS SPARE
_____ UNDERSTANDS STRIKE
_____ HELPS TO KEEP SCORE _____ WRITES NUMBERS _____ ADDS

Basketball Skills

_____ CAN CATCH ABOVE/BELOW WAIST
_____ PASSES
    _____ CHEST
    _____ BOUNCE
    _____ UNDERHAND
    _____ OVERHEAD
_____ CAN DRIBBLE WHILE STATIONARY
_____ CAN DRIBBLE WHILE WALKING
_____ CAN DRIBBLE WHILE RUNNING
_____ SHOTS
    _____ FREE THROW
    _____ CHEST/TWO-HAND
    _____ OVERHEAD
    _____ 1-HAND PUSH
_____ KNOWS HOW TO SCORE POINTS
_____ KNOWS WHAT A FOUL IS

_____ WILL GUARD AN OPPONENT
_____ WILL PASS TO A TEAMMATE
_____ WILL RECEIVE A PASS FROM TEAMMATE

Softball (Kickball—Tee Ball) Skills

_____ THROWS _____ OVERHAND _____ UNDERHAND
_____ CATCHES ABOVE THE WAIST WITH HANDS
_____ CATCHES BELOW THE WAIST WITH HANDS
_____ CATCHES WITH A GLOVE
_____ HOLDS A BAT CORRECTLY
_____ HAS PROPER BATTING STANCE
_____ SWINGS BAT WITH FOLLOW THROUGH/WEIGHT SHIFT
_____ HITS BALL AND RUNS TO FIRST BASE
_____ KNOWS BASE NAMES/RUNS THEM IN ORDER
_____ KNOWS CONCEPT OF "SAFE" AND "OUT"
_____ KNOWS WHEN TO ADVANCE ON THE BASES
_____ UNDERSTANDS STRIKE OUT _____ FLY OUT _____ TAG OUT
_____ FORCE OUT
_____ KNOWS HOW TO FIELD A BALL AND THROW TO A BASEMAN

Kickball

_____ WILL KICK BALL AND RUN TO THE BASES

Tee Ball

_____ WILL HIT BALL OFF THE TEE AND RUN THE BASES

Volleyball Skills

_____ CAN HIT A BALL OVERHEAD
_____ CAN SERVE THE BALL UNDERHAND
_____ CAN SERVE OVERHAND
_____ WILL ATTEMPT A "BUMP" SHOT
_____ HITS BALL OVER THE NET
_____ SERVES AND MOVES BACK INTO PLAYING AREA
_____ UNDERSTANDS 3 HITS TO A SIDE
_____ UNDERSTANDS BOUNDARY LINES/NET BOUNDARIES
_____ UNDERSTANDS ROTATION/MOVES WHEN GIVEN INSTRUCTION

Soccer Skills

_____ DRIBBLES BALL IN A STRAIGHT LINE
_____ DRIBBLES BALL AROUND OBSTACLES
_____ PASSES BALL TO TEAMMATE
_____ KICKS FOR GOAL
_____ STOPS BALL WITH FOOT _____ KNEE _____ CHEST

_____ CAN DEFEND HIS/HER GOAL
_____ GUARDS OPPONENTS
_____ ONLY USES FEET
_____ RECEIVES PASS AND SHOOTS FOR GOAL
_____ UNDERSTANDS GOALKEEPER'S POSITION

Touch Football Skills

_____ CAN CATCH A PASS ABOVE THE WAIST _____ BELOW THE WAIST
_____ CAN CATCH A PASS WHILE STATIONARY _____ WHILE MOVING
_____ CAN CATCH A PUNTED BALL
_____ THROWS A FORWARD PASS
_____ PUNTS
_____ PLACE KICKS
_____ KNOWS HOW TO BLOCK THE OPPOSITE TEAM WITH FOLDED ARMS
_____ WILL TRY TO RUN FOR A TOUCHDOWN
_____ KNOWS WHEN TO HUDDLE
_____ UNDERSTANDS HOW TO "TOUCH" PLAY WITH THE BALL
_____ UNDERSTANDS HOW TO GET "FLAG" OFF IN FLAG FOOTBALL
_____ UNDERSTANDS PLAY STOPS WHEN RUNNER IS TOUCHED OR FLAGGED

Floor Hockey Skills

_____ CAN HIT PUCK TO PARTNER
_____ STOPS PUCK HIT TO HIM/HER
_____ DRIBBLES PUCK
_____ UNDERSTANDS HOW TO SHOOT FOR GOAL AND SCORE POINTS
_____ PASSES PUCK/BALL TO TEAMMATE
_____ RECEIVES PASSES AND SHOOTS FOR GOAL
_____ UNDERSTANDS CONCEPT OF GUARDING
_____ UNDERSTANDS DIFFERENCE IN DEFENDING OWN GOAL AND TRYING TO SCORE POINTS

Badminton Skills

_____ CAN HIT SMALL BALL WITH RACKET OVER THE NET
_____ CAN HIT BIRDIE WITH RACKET OVER THE NET
_____ CAN SERVE UNDERHAND
_____ CAN KEEP BIRDIE/BALL WITHIN BOUNDARIES
_____ KNOWS HOW TO SCORE POINTS
_____ CAN PLAY SINGLES/DOUBLES

Mini-Golf

_____ CAN SWING PUTTER PROPERLY
_____ CAN REGULATE FORCE OF PUTT

_____ COUNTS HITS TO HOLE
_____ STARTS PUTTING AT "TEE OFF"
_____ WAITS HIS/HER TURN

Appendix D

ADAPTED SPORTS RULES

Baseball

- The names of the bases are: Home, First, Second, Third. (Diagram the bases and have student name them.)
- When the ball is hit, run to first base; if no one has the ball, run to second, third, home.
- Stay on the base until the ball is hit again.
- Everytime someone runs around all the bases and crosses home base, it scores 1 run or point.
- In order to run, the ball must be hit (off a tee or from the pitcher) and stay inside the boundaries.
- Each batter gets 3 swings at the ball; if s/he misses, s/he is out and his/her turn is done.
- There are 3 outs for each side. When 3 outs are done, the batter's team and the pitcher's team change places.
- If a hit ball is caught on a fly before it hits the ground, it is an out and the turn is done.
- If a player with the ball tags the runner, the runner is out and the turn is done.
- The pitcher stands on the pitchers' mound and throws the ball for the batter to hit it.
- The game is _____ innings long, each team batting, Whoever has the most runs/points wins.

Basketball

- Each basket counts 2 points
- There are 2 baskets, one on each end of the court. One is your team's and the other is the other team's.
- The ball is moved by passing or dribbling.
- The ball may be taken from another player as long as the player is not touched.
- A game is played in 4 quarters (parts), with a rest in-between each one. Each part is _____ minutes long. (Decide how long each quarter should be depending on the age and skill of the students.) After 4 quarters are played, the game is over. Whoever has the most points wins.

Bowling:

- Roll the ball at the pins
- Stay behind the foul line
- If all the pins do not fall down on the first ball, a second is rolled; that is one turn.
- All 10 pins down with the first ball is a strike.
- All 10 pins down with 2 balls is a spare.
- A ball in the gutter counts as one turn.
- Write down or tell someone the number of pins down on each roll.
- Develop a modified scoring sheet.
- Just have the total number of pins down in the large part of the sheet. First ball can be scored in smaller area—then count total pins and record. Don't mark spares or strikes initially; after the student is able to write the numbers in correctly, allow him/her to mark X or / as needed.

Floor Hockey

- Object is to hit the puck through the goal.
- Only the hockey stick may be used to move the puck.
- Keep the puck in bounds to be fair.
- A point is scored when the puck is hit between cones.
- There are 2 goals, one at each end of the boundaries.
- Try to keep the other players from making a goal by using the stick to take the puck away.
- The game is played in two halves, _____ minutes long. At the end of the game, whoever has the most points wins.

Four-Square

- The object is to get no points.
- One person stands in each square.
- At least one foot must always be in the square.
- The ball is hit in an underhand manner, with 1 or 2 hands to any other player.
- The ball must bounce one time before that player may hit the ball.
- The ball cannot hit a line.
- Only the player who misses the ball gets points.
- After someone misses, players change squares.

Kickball

- Same basic rules as baseball—changes would be:
- The pitcher rolls the ball to the batter to kick.
- In order to run, the ball must be kicked and stay in bounds.

Soccer

- The object is to kick the ball through the goal.
- Only feet may be used to touch the ball—no hands.
- Kick the ball softly to move it.
- Keep the ball within the boundaries to be fair.
- A point is scored when the ball is kicked between the cones (or whatever goal is used).
- If hands are used, the other player/team gets to kick the ball.
- The game is played in 2 halves/parts, each _____ minutes long. At the end of the whole game, whoever has the most points wins.
- Try to keep the other players from scoring points.

Volleyball

- The ball must stay in the air.
- If the ball hits the floor, it is a point for the other person/team.
- One or two hands may be used to volley the ball.
- The ball should stay within the boundaries to be fair (mark lines on the floor with tape).
- Initially allow unlimited hits per person/per side, then gradually set limits (example: 5 hits per side or 2 times per person).
- Game is over when one team has 15 points.

Appendix E

TEACHING HINTS AND GYMNASIUM ACTIVITY AREAS

In addition to teaching the actual skills to the children, there are some techniques that may be helpful in enhancing the teaching. Some are as follows:

- When walking on a balance beam, you walk in front of the child, facing him/her. Have *them* hold onto a baton, bar, or cut broom handle which you rest in the palms of your hands. Let *them* hold it and experience the feeling of "falling" and catching their balance, rather than you guiding them.
- Begin teaching jumping in place, on mattress, mini-tramp or with a hippity-hop. This helps them feel the bending of their knees.
- Next help them to jump down. If the child needs assistance, stand facing the child and put your hands on his/her hips which is the center of gravity. Tell the child "jump" and tip the child forward so his balance is moved ahead and he begins to "fall-jump." He may place his hands on your arms. As he falls, allow his weight to pull him down; support him only on the landing. As the child falls forward, you take a step back and say, "Jump down."
- Jumping up and over is best done with rope or string in a higher and lower manner.
- Jumping over or out is difficult for children who have motor problems. This is because not only do they have to get their body up, they also have to move it out. Use carpet squares, hoops, or mark a spot on the floor to which the child is to jump. This gives him a concrete place to go. If he needs help, stand behind him, hands on his hips, force him to bend his knees and then lift him up and out to the next square.
- To encourage long jumping, once the child is able to jump forward, use a variety of different-sized carpet squares, pieces of paper, etc., as indicators of distance. For instance, I have carpet squares 6″, 13″, and 28″ wide, plus one that is 32″ long. They are very handy.
- Modified hopscotch is played by initially just jumping square to square and not doing any hopping as in regular hopscotch. Once the child can hop, she can play normally.
- When *teaching* ball skills, work on one skill at a time, even though they are combined, i.e., catch and toss. That way you don't become as confused with praise and instruction.
- Use carpet squares, hoops, marks on the floor again to help the child understand where she is supposed to stand/sit and remain. Many times a child will

110

walk toward you on each toss. This eliminates the need to reposition the child after each toss, roll, kick, etc.

- It is also best to have a number of balls for immediate use rather than only one or two. This eliminates having to chase balls as they roll away.
- Many times physical assistance is necessary initially to help the child understand the movement. Stand behind the child to assist them through the movement.
- Footprints help identify placement of feet for throwing.
- Bean bags are useful to keep balls still for kicking. Place the ball on the bean bag and it will not roll.
- Allow for as much independence as possible with each child. Build in successful activities for them while practicing skills.

throw

kick

GYM/ASSESSMENT ACTIVITY AREAS

SEPARATE AREAS
PER BALL SKILL-
LEARN ONE CONCEPT
AT A TIME
BEFORE COMBINING
SKILLS

catch

PLAY AREA - GROUP GAMES/MUSIC

ride   **big wheel**
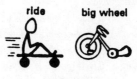

record player

roll

BALANCE, CLIMBING AND JUMPING ACTIVITIES

jungle gym   **slide**

jump   **climb**   **run**

OBSTACLE COURSES

Appendix F

RESOURCES AND MATERIALS ON AUTISM

Bacharach, A. W. *Developmental therapy for young children with autistic characteristics.* Baltimore: University Park Press, 1978.

Dalrymple, N. *Helping Children with autism manage their behavior.* Bloomington, Indiana: Indiana University Developmental Training Center, 1983.

Dalrymple, N. *Learning together.* Bloomington, Indiana: Indiana University Developmental Training Center, 1979.

Gilliam, J. E. (Ed.). *Autism, diagnosis, instruction, management, and research.* Springfield: Charles C Thomas, 1981.

Indiana University Developmental Training Center. *Educating Autistic/Severely Handicapped Children: Elementary Age.* Bloomington: Author et al., 1980.

Knoblock, P. *Teaching and mainstreaming autistic children.* Denver: Love Publishing Company, 1982.

Koegel, R. L. *How to integrate autistic and other severely handicapped children in a classroom.* Lawrence, KS: H & H Enterprises, Inc., 1982.

Koegel, R. L., Rincover, A., & Egel, A. L. *Educating and understanding autistic children.* San Diego: College-Hill, 1982.

McHale, S. M., Olley, J. G., Marcus, L. M., & Simeonsson, R. J. "Nonhandicapped peers as tutors for autistic children." *Exceptional Children,* 1981, 48(3), 263–265.

Park, C. C. "Elly and the right to education." *Phi Delta Kappan,* April 1974.

Russo, D. C., & Koegel, R. L. "A method for integrating an autistic child into a normal public school classroom." *Journal of Applied Behavior Analysis,* 1977, 10(4), 579–590.

Rutter, M. "Autism: educational issues." *Special Education,* September 1970.

Wing, L. *Children Apart: Autistic Children and Their Families,* Autism Society of America (ASA) Washington, DC, 1973.

Wing, L. *How They Grow: A handbook for parents of young children with autism,* National Society for Autistic Children (NSAC) Washington, DC.

Appendix G

RESOURCES AND MATERIALS ON GROSS MOTOR ASPECTS OF AUTISM

Best, J. F., and Jones, J. G. "Movement therapy in the treatment of autistic children." *Australian Occupational Therapy Journal,* 1974, 21(2) 72–86 (Journal published at Box 172, Subiaco, Western Australia 6008.)

Davis, D. H. "The balance beam: A bridge to cooperation." *Teaching Exceptional Children,* 1975, (3)94–95.

Dewey, M. "The autistic child in a physical education class." *Journal of Health, Physical Education, and Recreation,* 1972, 43(4): 79–80.

Dewey, M. *Recreation for autistic and emotionally disturbed children.* Rockville, MD.: National Institute of Mental Health. (ERIC Document Reproduction Service No. ED 094 495.)

Hamilton, A., Anderson, P., and Merton, K. "Learning to talk while developing motor skills." *Journal of Health, Physical Education, and Recreation,* 1972, 43(4):80–81.

Henn, J. M. *Adaptive physical education for the severely handicapped.* Bloomington, Indiana: Indiana University Developmental Training Center, 1978.

Henning, J. et al. *Teaching social and leisure skills to youth with autism.* Bloomington, Indiana: Indiana University Developmental Training Center, 1982.

Kraft, R. E. "Physical activity for the autistic child." *Physical Educator,* March 1983, 40(1): 33–37.

Mangus, B. C., & Henderson, H. "Providing physical education to autistic children." *Palaestra,* Winter, 1988, 4(2):38–43.

Mosher, R. "Perceptual-motor training and the autistic child." *Journal of Leisurability,* 1975, 2(3):29–25.

Ornitz, E. M., "The modulation of sensory input and motor output in autistic children." *Journal of Autism and Childhood Schizophrenia,* 1974, 4(3):197–215.

Reid, G., & Morin, B. "Physical education for autistic children." *Canadian Association for Health, Physical Education and Recreation Journal.* Sept–Oct 1981, 48(1):25–29.

Schleien, S. J., Heyne, L. A., Berken, S. B., "Integrating physical education to teach appropriate play skills to learners with autism." *Adapted Physical Activity Quarterly,* July 1988, 5(3):182–192.

Schmidt, G., McLaughlin, J., & Dalrymple, N. "Teaching students with autism. A sport skill specialist's approach." *Journal of Health, Physical Education, Recreation, and Dance,* Sept. 1986, 57(7):60–63.

Winnick, J. P., and Landus, D. M. "Try trampolining with handicapped children." *Teaching Exceptional Children,* summer 1971.

Physical Education and Related Programs for Autistic and Emotionally Disturbed Children, AAHPERD. 1976.

ADDITIONAL ASSESSMENT OPTIONS

AAHPER Special Fitness Test for Mildly Mentally Retarded Persons
Cratty Six Category Gross Motor Test
Godfrey-Kephart Movement Pattern Checklist Short Form
Purdue Perceptual Motor Survey
Vineland Adaptive Behavior Scales
HELP Hawaii Early Learning Profile (0–3)
Brigance Inventory of Early Development (0–7)

GLOSSARY

ADAPTED PHYSICAL EDUCATION—safe, successful gross motor activity time that is structured and has instruction.

AUTISM—severe developmental disability characterized by deficits in communication and social interaction, a restricted repertoire of activities and interests, and onset in infancy or early childhood.

APHASIA—a general impairment of language functioning, most often associated with cerebral palsy.

AUGMENTATIVE SYSTEMS—systems designed to enhance communication through means other than oral speech, examples might include communication boards or sign language.

ACADEMIC—school-type activities

ATTENTION SPAN—amount of time spent concentrating on a given activity.

COMMUNICATION IMPAIRED—difficulty in adequately expressing or comprehending daily communication.

COMMUNICATION BOARD—board or book used to communicate a message, which consists of pictures and/or written vocabulary that is accessed by point, eye gaze, or electronic switch.

COPING SKILLS—ability to interact in society and maintain a level of functionality.

CRITERION REFERENCED—test in which students are compared with a predetermined standard of performance rather than with others of their age.

CHARTING—maintaining a record of observable skills/behaviors over a specified period of time.

DSM III-R—Diagnostic and Statistical Manual, third edition, revised, of the American Psychiatric Association.

DEVELOPMENTAL HISTORY—written record obtained from parents/guardian regarding child's first 3 years specifically, to assist in the diagnosis of autism.

DEVELOPMENTAL PROFILE—chart of educational/functional skills scores from an interdisciplinary team assessment.

DEVELOPMENTAL MILESTONES—time in child's life when certain skills appear.

DESENSITIZATION—step-by-step reduction of anxiety associated with changes in routine, introduction of new people/stimuli, or changes in environment.

115

ECHOLALIA—the repetition of another's words or phrases either immediately or delayed. Can be used communicatively or can also be without apparent meaning.

EXPRESSIVE LANGUAGE—language that is directed to others which may be oral, written or through the use of augmentative systems.

FRAGILE X SYNDROME—genetic syndrome affecting males resulting from an abnormality on the X chromosome—associated with physical features such as protruding ears, large testicles, large head, elongated face and large hands and feet and with mental retardation and possible autism.

FUNCTIONAL SKILLS—repertoire of lifetime skills, such as eating, dressing, work-type activities

FRUSTRATORS—activities/objects/individuals that create anxiety and stress for people with autism.

GENERALIZATION—ability of learning one skill and relating it to the learning of another.

GROSS MOTOR—large muscle play activities, running, jumping, ball skills.

HIGH FUNCTIONING CHILDREN WITH AUTISM—child with autism who is not also retarded.

HYPOREACTIVE—under-sensitivity to stimuli

HYPERREACTIVE—over-sensitivity to stimuli

INTERDISCIPLINARY—group of professionals from various disciplines working together in a cooperative fashion.

INTERDISCIPLINARY ASSESSMENT—evaluation completed by an interdisciplinary team who work together, often simultaneously, observing each other's activities in order to enhance the total picture of the child.

INFORMATION–SHARING MEETING—post-assessment exchange of assessment results among interdisciplinary team.

IEP—individualized education plan which is required by law for all children with disabilities. It includes the goals and objectives for the student that are planned by teachers, parents, and support staff according to the child's needs.

LOW FUNCTIONING CHILDREN WITH AUTISM—children who are retarded along with having autism.

LANGUAGE/COMMUNICATION—ability to express oneself and to understand others.

LD—learning disabled

LRE—least restrictive environment, the most "normal" environment that can be provided for a child with disabilities.

LESSON PLAN—daily schedule of activities

MENTAL RETARDATION—significant subaverage general intellectual functioning in certain individuals.

MILDLY MENTALLY RETARDED—degree of retardation with the range of intelligence scores of 50–55 to 70.

MODERATELY MENTALLY RETARDED—degree of retardation with the range of intelligence scores of 35–40 to 50 or 55.

MOTIVATORS—activities/objects/people which entice students to work.

MINIMAL ASSISTANCE—least amount of physical guidance necessary to complete an activity.

NONVERBAL TESTING—testing in which no or minimal verbal directions or responses are required. Results are based on observing and reproducing desired response techniques.

NEXT STEPS—activities that are appropriate follow up for students' skill level.

OBSERVATIONAL CHECKLIST—organized list of skills that child may perform during an assessment period.

OBJECT ATTACHMENT—inappropriate clinging or need for certain objects, e.g., stuffed animal, strings, beads, in order to feel safe.

PL 94-142—Education for All Handicapped Children Act of U.S. Congress which mandates free, equal, and appropriate education for all children.

PKU—genetic disease caused by the absence of an enzyme that is necessary for the metabolism of the essential amino acid, phenylalanine. Can be treated if recognized early; babies are routinely screened within seven days of birth.

PREDICTABILITY—ability to know and rely on what will happen next, i.e., routine.

PLAY—free time activity

PEOPLE CENTERED—focus on people/examiners rather than activities or tasks.

PEP—psychoeducational profile, evaluation specifically designed for children with autism based on finding strengths as well as deficits.

PROBLEM SOLVING—ability to resolve conflict that may impede educational/play progress

RECEPTIVE LANGUAGE—ability to understand written, verbal, or assisted communication

SCHEDULE BOOK—individualized book that contains symbols, pictures, or words pertaining to a student's day.

SOCIAL—interactions with others.

SELF-HELP—skills of daily living such as eating, dressing, toileting, bathing, etc.

SIGN LANGUAGE—a communication system that utilizes gestures, finger spelling, or signing.

SELF-STIMULATION—use of body, objects, music, or other material/sounds to calm or excite oneself.

SELF-ABUSE—hurting oneself.

STANDARDIZED ASSESSMENT—evaluations that have specifics as to directions, activities and administration. Data has been established on reliability and norms.

SEVERE/PROFOUND MENTAL RETARDATION—degree of retardation with a range of intelligence scores of below 20–25 to 35–40.

SPLINTER SKILLS—segments of larger skills, e.g., excellent ability to memorize facts without the ability to use the facts functionally.

TOTAL ASSISTANCE—complete physical guidance needed to complete an activity.

TASK CENTERED—focus on activities of an assessment rather than on the examiner.

VINELAND—a rating scale of adaptive behaviors.

VERBAL TESTING—assessments that involve the use of language to instruct and/or respond.

BIBLIOGRAPHY

Coleman, M., and Gillberg, C.: *The biology of autistic syndromes.* New York, Praeger, 1985.

DeMyer, M.: *Parents and children in autism.* Washington D.C., Winston and Sons, 1979.

Felicetti, T.: "Parents of autistic children: some notes on a chemical connection." *Milieu Therapy, 1:*13–16, 1981.

Gillberg, C.: "Brief Report: Onset at age 14 of a typical autistic syndrome. A case report of a girl with Herpes Simplex Encephalitis." *Journal of Autism and Developmental Disabilities, 16:*369–375, 1986.

Gillberg, C.: "Infantile autism and other childhood psychoses in a Swedish urban region. Epidemiological aspects." *Journal of Child Psychology and Psychiatry, 25:*35–43, 1984.

Langendorfer, S.: "Label motor patterns, not kids: A developmental perspective for adapted physical education." *Physical Educator,* Early winter, 1985.

Levy, S.: personal communication, 1986.

Levy, S., Mecca, A. and Porco, B.: personal communications as part of the Autism Training Team at the Institute for the Study of Developmental Disabilities, Indiana University, 1986.

Prizant, B., and Schuler, A.: "Facilitating Communication: Language Approaches." In *Handbook on autism and pervasive developmental disorders.* New York, Wiley, 1987.

Ritvo, E., and Freeman, B. J.: *Diagnosis and Definition of Autism.* National Society for Children with Autism, 1978.

Rutter, M.: "Cognitive deficits in the pathogenesis of autism." *Journal of Child Psychology and Psychiatry, 24:*513–531, 1983.

Wing, L.: *Early Childhood Autism* (2nd ed.). Oxford, Pergamon, 1980.

Wing, L., and Gould, J.: "Severe impairments of social interaction and associated abnormalities in children: Epidemiology and classification." *Journal of Autism and Developmental Disorders, 9:*11–29, 1979.

INDEX